A Passion for Living

A Passion for Living

*The amazing story of a boy
who makes every day matter*

ALEXANDER STOBBS

HODDER

First published in Great Britain in 2009 by Hodder & Stoughton
An Hachette UK company

First published in paperback in 2010

I

Copyright © Alexander Stobbs 2009

A CIP catalogue record for this title
is available from the British Library

ISBN 978 0 340 97853 5

Typeset in Plantin Light by Ellipsis Books Limited, Glasgow

Printed and bound by Clays Ltd, St Ives plc

To my family, and the fantastic staff at
the Royal Brompton Hospital who've managed
to put up with me for over nineteen years.

Contents

Acknowledgements

Grateful thanks to my mum and dad who encouraged me to write, to Judith Longman at Hodder and to Caro Handley, who kept me in check, and lastly, Ralph Allwood who has forever been supportive.

Introduction

by Alex Stobbs

When *A Boy Called Alex* was shown on Channel 4 early in 2008, I didn't expect anything other than a few kind words from family and friends. So I was overwhelmed and very touched when I received literally hundreds of emails and letters from people all over the world. Some of them simply said 'well done', while others were from people facing challenges of their own, who said I'd given them encouragement and hope. I got stopped in the street many times – I still do – by people saying 'you're the kid from the documentary, aren't you?', or 'you're the conductor' and they always had something kind to say.

Some of the letters were from musicians offering to take part in my next project. At the end of the film, which told the story of my quest to conduct Bach's *Magnificat*, I was asked what I wanted to do next. That was a pretty straightforward one for me, as I'd already thought about it many times. I replied, 'Bach's *St Matthew Passion* – all three hours of it.' I knew it was a huge undertaking, but I felt I could do it. I didn't want to settle for a shorter or simpler work, because the *Matthew Passion* means so much to me – it is one of the most wonderful, dramatic and inspiring pieces of music ever written, and I knew I just had to have the chance to conduct it. When professional musicians wrote to say they would like to take part, I felt incredibly moved by their generosity and encouragement.

This book covers the year from April 2008 up to 5 April 2009, when I fulfilled that dream by conducting the *Matthew Passion* at Cadogan Hall in London. It was one of the most important years of my life, because not only was I planning to conduct the *Passion*, but I was also taking my A levels, leaving school, and starting my university degree – studying music at Cambridge.

Along the way I had some pretty tough times. I was ill during my A levels, and then just before going to university I had to go into hospital for a couple of weeks, and I was back there again for another three weeks a few days after I arrived in Cambridge. That was a big low; I was pretty ill and I felt desperate about missing the start of my first term. But I made up for lost time when I got back, and there have been some real highs during the year – mostly through people who have been supportive and believed in me. I have certainly come to realise what good friends I have, and I've also made some incredible new ones.

Introduction

Cystic fibrosis (often abbreviated to CF) is a pretty annoying disease – I wouldn't wish it on anyone. That's why it means a great deal to me to encourage awareness of it, and support research. That, more than anything else, is what made me decide to write this book. I want people to know about CF, and I hope very much that some people reading it will want to help – either by giving towards research, or perhaps just by telling others more about the condition.

CF is the most common life-threatening inherited disease in the UK. One in every 2,500 babies is born with it, and there are currently 7,500 people who have it. But wonderful, pioneering work is being done. In the 1960s, few children with CF lived beyond the age of ten. Today, most people make it to thirty, and some will live to forty. That's real progress and worth celebrating, but there's still a long way to go, and I very much hope that, in some small way, this book will help.

It's never easy talking about what it's like to have CF. In fact, I've spent most of my time trying to ignore it and simply getting on with my life, so having to sit and write about what it feels like, and the part it plays in my life, hasn't been easy. But I wanted to do it because I've found myself in the position of being in the public eye, so I can talk about it on behalf of the many others who are dealing with the same problems.

Like a lot of other people who live with ill health, I'm quite driven, determined and – dare I say it – very stubborn at times. My mum always says I push myself too hard (and she's probably right), but I have always seen difficult things as a challenge rather than an obstacle, and I just have to prove myself. Nothing gives me more satisfaction than being able to say 'I did it' and prove the doubters wrong. I'm not the kind of person to be cautious or give in; I want to show others that having CF doesn't mean sitting around feeling sorry for yourself. I'd much rather be striving to achieve things than dwelling on the downside of it all.

I want to thank all the people who have helped me throughout my journey so far. The many doctors and nurses in London, Cambridge and Kent who have got me back on my feet time after time, the teachers who have encouraged me, and the friends who cracked gags when I needed them most, and who have never viewed me as someone who is 'ill'. Most of all, though, I want to thank my family, who have always put me first, loved me no matter how annoying I have been, and taught me that no obstacle is ever too big.

A Mother's Story

by *Suzanne Stobbs*

Of the many hospital appointments I have been to with Alexander, my son, the one following his sixth birthday stands out quite clearly in my mind. It was in our local hospital at Pembury, in Kent. As we opened the consulting room door, Alexander's kindly paediatrician, Dr Joe Meyer, swung round in his chair, smiled at us, and said, 'Six last week, Alexander. How time flies!'

Alexander grinned, but my immediate response was 'Actually, no, it has seemed more like sixty'. Dr Meyer raised his eyebrows in a quizzical fashion, then smiled in empathy as I sank gratefully down, into one of the large chairs by his desk.

The years since Alexander's birth had been effervescent with activity. Apart from coping with the usual demands of four young children born in quick succession, I was home-schooling two of them, driving long distances to take my daughter to her prep school, keeping an eye on elderly parents, *and* trying to get to grips with Alexander's complex medical needs. Days and nights often coalesced as I attempted to catch up with household chores, repeatedly interrupted by Alexander's coughing fits and bouts of sickness. And then there were the dreaded midnight drugs. Little wonder that time could seem suspended; caught in a never-ending sea of need and want that in ensuing years would show no change.

Alexander is the youngest of my four and was born on 30 January 1990, two weeks early, with the umbilical cord wrapped twice around his neck. I recall the midwife's momentary look of alarm, before she swiftly and expertly cut the cord. He was the smallest and lightest of my children, weighing little more than six pounds, and I remember thinking how fragile he looked, and so very pale; a living porcelain doll with a light crown of fine dark hair and unusually sad and forlorn eyes.

Right from the start, breastfeeding proved difficult. I had had no problems at all with the other three, but as I tried to feed Alexander he would become tetchy and fretful, greedy for milk, but unable to suckle for long, drawing up his legs in obvious discomfort as colicky pain set in. What little milk he did take in would be quickly regurgitated – and then the pitiful wails of hunger would begin all over again.

The nursing staff in the hospital where he was born were naturally concerned, not only because of

Alexander's poor feeding pattern, but because he had failed to pass meconium, which are the bright green stools of newborn babies, normally excreted soon after birth. (I later learned that 10 to 15 per cent of babies with cystic fibrosis (CF) show intestinal obstruction within twenty-four hours of birth.) As a result, my intended overnight stay turned into several days and nights.

Meanwhile, my husband, Tim, was holding the fort at home. Thankfully, our daughter Miranda, who was by now four and a half, had just started school. Three-year-old Christian attended playgroup a couple of mornings a week, and Patrick, a year younger, was the only one needing twenty-four-hour supervision.

Within a day or so Alexander had passed the meconium and his feeding became more settled, so to our relief – and the delight of his two brothers and sister – he was finally discharged. I was advised, though, to go straight to my GP if I had any cause for concern.

By this time Alexander weighed less than he had done at birth, and because he was so tiny I had very few Babygros that fitted him, so one of my first trips out was to drive to our local town, Tunbridge Wells, to buy a good supply of clothes in premature-baby sizes. I remember thinking how nice it was for him to have something brand-new, and not handed down from the other three.

As the days passed and Tim returned to his daily commute to London, I began to get back to my normal routine: ferrying the children to school and playgroup, accompanied by Alexander in a brand-new portable car seat, lined with a super-soft sheepskin rug to keep his tiny frame warm.

I loved every minute of being with the children and felt very happy. My only slight niggle was that feeding times continued to be difficult, with Alexander still tending to regurgitate his milk, sometimes with projectile force and often with a curious rattle. I was breastfeeding on demand, and with his stomach never sufficiently full, I had to have him with me all the time. I enjoyed breastfeeding, but the sickness and frequency with which I had to change his clothes and bedding was wearying. I also noticed how quickly the milk shot through his system, and that he needed changing almost continuously. At this point I rang both a nutritionist and a breastfeeding counsellor for advice. But, like my own GP, they didn't seem unduly concerned and their advice was to give the situation more time to settle.

A health check at two weeks revealed that Alexander was still not back up to his birth weight, and he remained extremely pale. His skin was translucent, almost ethereal, and had a curious mottled pattern. But my health visitor, Marie-Louise Glover (who was herself to have a baby with CF a few years later), visited us regularly and so, with a new house and our other three children to look after as well, I pushed my worries to the back of my mind.

But when Alexander was seven weeks old, life suddenly took on a new urgency following a routine visit to our local health clinic. Compared to the plump, rosy-hued, lusty-lunged babies that filled the room, I was struck by Alexander's frail physique and pallor. Totally unresponsive to the cries of the babies around him, he almost looked as though he had given up on life, resigned and still.

Marie-Louise, who was supervising that particular clinic, took one look at him that day and immediately telephoned the paediatric ward in Pembury, telling them to expect a baby who she suspected could be quite seriously ill. It was then, very gently, she voiced her concerns to me that she thought Alexander might have some sort of metabolic disorder.

My initial feeling was one of relief that Alexander was going to be taken off my hands and sorted out. In my ignorance, a metabolic disorder suggested some allergy or other treatable condition. It didn't cross my mind that it might be something more serious, let alone a life-threatening disease. So, having asked a close friend to look after the other children until Tim got back from London, I set off for the hospital with Alexander and Marie-Louise.

On arrival at the hospital, Alexander was examined by a number of doctors. Initially, they wanted to rule out pyloric stenosis, a congenital condition in which the lower part of the stomach is narrowed, causing a violent spasm of vomiting, because the food is unable to get through to the small intestine. When they were babies, both Tim and his brother John had had the necessary surgery for this complaint, and we all hoped that this would be the diagnosis – an easily cured condition that would happily end all of Alexander's troubles. However, this was quickly ruled out and a nurse told me that they needed to do further tests to establish whether or not he had CF.

I remember going very quiet. The light surrounding Alexander's newborn presence, and which I cherished so much, had suddenly dimmed, and within the shadows I gradually began to under-stand what was really wrong with him. For I knew a little about CF, and I knew that Alexander was now facing a likely diagnosis of a life-threatening disease for which there was no cure.

I felt completely unprepared for this – not for one moment had I thought I'd find myself as the mother of a baby with a serious illness. I'd had no concerns with my other three, and my own mother had given birth to *seven* very healthy babies, including twins – of whom I am the youngest.

The news was then broken to us that Alexander needed to be admitted to hospital. And, fearing this could be a lengthy stay, Tim rang his mother to ask if she could come and look after our other children, which she very kindly did.

Alexander was immediately put on a saline and dextrose drip to help rehydrate him. By now he seemed to be visibly deteriorating in front of our eyes. It was just so distressing seeing him in such obvious pain as the nursing staff attempted to insert needles carrying the vital liquid into his sparrow-like arms. (It was probably just as well that we didn't know then that over the next few years this was a scene to be repeated a hundred or more times.)

He was then subjected to a number of investigations, including blood tests, chest X-rays and stool collections. The most significant test, though, would be the sweat test. This is a key indicator of CF, as those with the condition have an increased amount of salt in their sweat due to irregular salt flow in the body's cells. In fact, my health visitor had already asked me if I had noticed a salty taste when kissing Alexander and I had replied that I had – little realising the awful significance of this.

On the morning of the sweat test I refused to accompany Alexander to the treatment room, where they were going to swaddle his right arm in layers of plastic wadding in order to promote a good amount of sweat. I felt that I just could not be complicit in what might be the final diagnosis of a disease that causes tremendous suffering and early death. It was with incredible angst that I watched him as he lay cradled in the nurse's arms as he was being taken away.

That day, Tim had brought Christian and Patrick

into the hospital to see their little brother. It was a beautiful spring morning in March and, having collected Alexander from the treatment room, we sat outside the League of Friends shop, feeling slightly better for a dose of sunshine and the boys for a good helping of chocolate – the two of them blissfully unaware of the morning's horrendous significance.

I felt hollow still and quietly reflective. Deep down I knew what the diagnosis would be, but awaited the confirmation with reservation and anxiety.

When the results finally came through, Dr Meyer gently relayed the findings: Alexander did indeed have CF. It was not a good diagnosis, he said, but statistics showed that babies, children and even young adults with the disease were doing better all the time. There was, he added, every reason to be positive and optimistic.

Although Dr Meyer meant well, his words of hope were lost on me. Tim, as ever, remained positive – but then he knew nothing of my early friendship with a girl who had suffered from the disease. I had seen CF ravage her body, and in her last year of life she had become crippled, reliant on oxygen, and needing twenty-four-hour care, which was given unstintingly by her loving parents.

She was an extraordinary person. Her serenity, compassion and warmth towards all those around her was deeply humbling. In her short life she never once complained about her illness and stoically accepted her treatments, however painful and exhausting. I recall her swallowing an inordinate number of pills, in between coughing up quantities of purulent green sputum, her body wracked by paroxysms of coughing. Movingly, she married her childhood sweetheart, but sadly died shortly afterwards.

By coincidence, my twin brother, Mark, had a year earlier become godfather to a child with CF; and, recalling my friend's awful struggle with the disease, I remember thinking about the difficult times that awaited him.

The faulty gene that causes CF can be found in one in twenty-five people, and if both parents are carriers, then the odds of them having a baby with CF is one in four.

Until Alexander was diagnosed, Tim and I had no idea we were both carriers, and it was only then that we realised how fortunate we had been to have already had three healthy children. We later met families with two, or even three, children with the disease.

CF mainly affects the lungs, digestive system and sweat glands. As I mentioned just now, it is a condition in which the body struggles to regulate the flow of salt between cells in organs, including the lungs, digestive system and pancreas. This altered flow of salt affects the production of digestive juices and so the food cannot be absorbed properly, leading to poor weight gain. The body's mucus is severely thickened as well, so that instead of protecting tissues from harm, as it should, it obstructs the ducts and airways, causing tissue damage and making the respiratory passages within the lungs more susceptible to bacterial infection. For this reason, frequent chest infections and poor digestion are the common complaints of CF sufferers, with resultant poor growth and complications such as osteoporosis, liver damage, diabetes and infertility.

Alexander, we later discovered, had the most common CF mutation, Delta F508. Life expectancy is uncertain, but on average a baby born in the 1990s would expect to live into their thirties. Most could expect frequent hospital admissions, regular courses of intravenous antibiotics to combat the lung infections, and need additional nutrition, including high-calorie supplements, or even enteral feeding by way of a gastrostomy. This is a permanent opening into the stomach to receive feeds, along with massive amounts of medication – including enzymes, steroids, antibiotics, vitamins, minerals, antacids, antifungal agents, puffers and nebulisers. As the lungs of those with CF get progressively worse, they also need the use of portable oxygen to assist breathing.

CF is a multi-system disease, involving multi-disciplinary medical teams. It carries with it an extraordinary workload which, in our case, would soon become all too apparent.

During Alexander's first week or so in hospital,

Tim and I were visited by a number of support teams, including physiotherapists, dieticians, social workers and psychologists. There was a huge amount to learn and we were deluged by books, pamphlets, leaflets and a whole array of goodies, including many freebie trial packs, which all seemed a little overwhelming.

Kind friends sent cards, baked cakes, and helped out generously with the care of our other children. One most welcome gift was a complete set of toy musical instruments ranging from chime bars to shakers and whistles which, as well as amusing the other three children, ended up being a stimulus for Alexander's early musical interest.

He was by now being given all the necessary medication vital for his illness, which was mainly crushed-up tablets and liquids taken with my breast milk, but he remained on a drip for several days. Thankfully, the nurses gently coaxed me through the difficult task of getting him to swallow the medication, and soon I began to feel a little less nervous about it all.

One day I had a visit from a friend, a former nurse who had not yet been told about Alexander's diagnosis. As I told her he had CF, she began to cry. 'It's such an awful illness,' she wailed.

Her reaction shook me. I felt quite indignant that anybody should feel so negative about such a young life, and I think it was in that split second that I made up my mind that I would do everything I possibly could to make Alexander's life a wonderful one. As the days went by Tim and I found ourselves completely united in our refusal to accept anything less than a truly positive outcome for Alexander, regardless of the diagnosis. His life, we agreed, would become a cause for celebration, not a lament for what might have been.

Of course, this positive front was hard to maintain all the time. The first Sunday following Alexander's diagnosis was Mothering Sunday, normally a day of celebration. But that year, with Alexander still in hospital, there was a feeling of deep poignancy about it. So, in need of support and company from my church friends and having settled Alexander after being with him overnight in hospital, I decided to drive the few miles to Brenchley church. It was only as I pulled up outside that I remembered the clocks had gone forward an hour, heralding the start of British Summertime. From my parked car, I watched the congregation streaming out of the church, clutching their pretty Mothering Sunday flower posies.

As one friend walked towards me, her daughter, on seeing my eyes fill with tears, thrust her flowers into my hands – a gesture of incredible kindness and one that was so hard to take. More tears came thick and fast as seven weeks of physical and mental exhaustion finally caught up with me.

Several months before Alexander was born, we had moved from a tiny converted cowshed to one-half of a pretty, chocolate-box Kent oast house, set within a small working fruit farm, formerly a hop farm, and surrounded on all sides by orchards with fields of cherries, plums, apples and pears spreading out into the distance. Half of this double-cowled oast was derelict and inhabited by mice and bats, while our side had been converted in the 1970s and was now badly in need of some TLC (though we neither had the time nor the funds to do anything about it).

From our oast roof we had a panoramic view across miles of orchards and fields of sheep, with the white shiny cowls of other oast houses nestling in the dips. Summer days saw the skies weighed down with hot-air balloons, moving majestically high above us. Periodically they landed in the field next door, much to the delight of the children.

The orchards, haystacks, the old hop poles, the derelict farm buildings, rusty oil cans, apple boxes and all the paraphernalia of a bygone age gave the children endless hours of pleasure and I used to let them roam free. Their resourcefulness in always finding something to amuse themselves with was a blessing as it let me concentrate on giving Alexander the attention he needed.

When his final discharge date was mooted, I set about spring cleaning our home with a vengeance. The carpets were cleaned, rugs beaten, curtains washed, and furniture dusted until the wood shone. Tim and I knew we simply had to be realistic about our situation. We had just moved into a rather shabby but beautiful house, situated in a truly picturesque spot, presenting a wonderful playground for the children. And, despite our worries about mud, dust, fleas, lice and even crop sprays, we knew we couldn't wrap Alexander in cotton wool. We simply had to make the best of our home situation.

In order to keep Alexander's medicines away from the other children I cleared out a cupboard set high in our little kitchen. And so began the 'Highlands Oast Pharmacy', which in future would take over two more cupboards, a whole new fridge, half the garage, and a big chunk of Alexander's room.

Soon my notice board was crammed with lists – from the amount of medication that Alexander was taking, to the times he should take it, to the next clinic appointment, health care checks, and all his prescription renewals. Not to mention, of course, the other children's school and playgroup events. Thankfully, Marie-Louise went out of her way to support me during those early post-hospital days, as I faced the difficult task of getting Alexander to swallow all his medication. Teaspoons of jam and fromage frais became the easiest way to get him to ingest the many multi-coloured pills that he needed. More often than not, though, he would spit or vomit them out – and if some did make their way in, the strong enzyme powder he needed would often ulcerate his mouth. Some of this powder would inevitably be transferred on to me, making feeding times painful for both of us.

Because Alexander's weight was still only increasing at a snail's pace, I agreed – reluctantly – to supplement his breast milk with bottles of full-cream cow's milk combined with large amounts of high-calorie powder. This was to be his staple diet for the next six years, although at times he had to be fed through a naso-gastric tube, passed up his nose and down into his stomach. This is an unpleasant procedure, but vital at times to maintain his weight.

Wherever we went, bottles of milk and the special powdered Duocal, together with tubs of fromage frais, accompanied us. For a long time that was all Alexander would eat, until at the age of three he started to accept spaghetti hoops and then gradually, over the next few years, he began to tackle home-made beef stew, crisps (always smoky bacon), ice-cream, Twix bars, strawberry milkshakes and McDonalds chicken nuggets and chips.

For some reason he did not want to eat food offered by other people, and this was a problem. At parties, as he got older, he would eat virtually nothing and was reluctant even to drink a prepared milkshake. Babies and children with CF are often reluctant eaters, but Alexander seemed so incredibly faddy about his food that, with hindsight, I think he should have been seen by an eating disorder specialist. However, the dieticians seemed happy enough with his gradual weight gain.

To fight off the fatigue that inevitably crept up on me during the day, I used to lie down with the children after lunch, sneaking off after twenty minutes to start the household chores. I did the same in the evening. Alexander was still prone to tummy ache and wind, with occasional bouts of sickness, and needing to have his back gently rubbed to placate him. But as I often fell asleep myself, I had to set an alarm. Late in the evening I became a night owl, using the little time I had to myself to make curtains and furnishings for the house.

Twice-daily sessions of physiotherapy were vital to keep Alexander's lungs healthy, by dislodging the pockets of mucus that are often prevalent in early chest infections. When he was a baby we could gently tap his chest. As a toddler, a physiotherapy bed or a foam wedge tipped him up for a more rigorous percussion.

Physiotherapy became increasingly important when, at eighteen months, Alexander's sputum revealed a significant growth of pseudomonas, a germ more usually associated with teenagers and young adults with CF. With this germ already in his lungs at such a young age, it was decided that he should have daily doses of antibiotics via a nebuliser. Soon steroids were introduced into the regime to fight inflammation, and various puffers used to open up his airways. By now, the 'Highlands Oast Pharmacy' was bursting at the seams.

After this Alexander became a regular in-patient at Pembury Hospital, having two-week courses of intravenous drugs, either infused or injected into cannulae inserted gently into his arms. As we lived only a twenty-minute drive away, it was easy to come and go with the other children in tow, and the hospital playroom became as much a home to his brothers and sister as it was to Alexander. Because it was a general paediatric unit, we encountered children and babies suffering from a variety of medical conditions – and from time to time we got a sharp reminder that life could deal out a very cruel set of cards.

On one occasion when we were in the playroom with Alexander, by now an agile, lively toddler, in walked one of Miranda's school friends and his mother. This little boy was having difficulty walking and, following tests, it was discovered he had an inoperable brain tumour. His death a couple of years later, at the age of just six, affected us all very deeply.

On the whole Alexander slotted well into his hospital home, happily vaulting off his high-sided cot and running down the shiny corridor to peep in at the nurses' office and other children's rooms. He was very much an 'on the go' happy child, full of smiles and laughter and generally accepting of his lot in life. The nurses loved him, but I found it terribly difficult leaving him there when I went home. I have often thought that the roads to Pembury, the A21 and, then later, the M25 and M11 must have been awash with my tears.

We joined our local CF support group and our meetings became focused not only on mutual support, but on raising awareness of the disease with a variety of fund-raising ventures. Tim and I, plus all four children, helped with house-to-house and street collections and often collected money outside shops, sometimes dressed in brightly coloured clown outfits. We also supported plant sales, fairs, concerts and sporting events. All the schools that Alexander went to were good at raising money for the Cystic Fibrosis Trust and numerous collections were taken at chapel services. Many years down the line, Tim was to run the London Marathon, at the age of fifty, in two hours fifty-nine minutes, coming thirty-fifth in his age group and raising over £7,000 for the Trust.

In the September following his fourth birthday, Alexander started school. All our children had begun at the local primary school, though the other three were no longer there, as Miranda had just gained an all-round award to a prep school and I had taken Patrick and Christian out of school in order to home-tutor them. Home education had always intrigued me and I felt that I could offer a good broadly based curriculum, with lots of trips out, free from any rigorous academic restraint – including all those tests!

Alexander, we felt, should initially go to our local

primary school, as the others had done, to establish good friendships. I had no worries about him fitting in as he was a gregarious child, full of fun and mischief, and he often had us in stitches. Academically he appeared strong and was a fluent reader, but health-wise I was worried. Coughs and colds, sore throats and viruses were all likely to be brought into the classroom. Games and long playground sessions might tire him out, and I knew that he wouldn't eat school lunch. In the end I compromised, letting him enjoy the rough and tumble with his peer group in the play-ground, but taking him home at lunchtime to eat.

By now music was filling our home. I was teaching the boys to play the piano and helping Miranda with her practice, and all four were having violin lessons in East Peckham with a wonderful lady called Frances Clack.

While Christian, Patrick and Miranda made good, steady progress in both their instruments, Alexander seemed to come on in leaps and bounds. He displayed a real gift and feel for music, and by the age of three he could play little pieces on the piano with both hands. He seemed to love it. I had bought him a portable music player, and he would drag this around the house in one hand, with a bottle of milk, or his small violin, in the other! He loved listening to the wonderful series called Classical Kids, which had been sent over from New Zealand by my sister, Jackie.

Christian and Patrick had joined Brenchley church

choir and enjoyed their singing so much that Tim and I decided to give them the option of becoming choristers. Christian won a place with Canterbury Cathedral Choir and Patrick at King's College Cambridge. These places came with the added bonus of substantially reduced prep school fees, but as choristers they had to board, and I found that very difficult. During their home-schooling years I had forged a special bond with both of them, and it was hard to let them go. And then, at just ten years old, and very determined to match her brothers' achievements, Miranda was also set to board after winning a music scholarship to Benenden.

With the other three away, I now had more time for Alexander, who naturally missed the company of his siblings. I was trying to think how best I could channel his obvious musical ability when I spotted an advertisement in our local paper for Stoke Brunswick School, in West Sussex, offering academic and music awards for talented children. I attended one of their open days and listened to the award-winning choir perform. I was spellbound and decided to enter Alexander for one of the awards, which he gained shortly after his seventh birthday on account, not only of his academic and musical ability but, as the headmaster later told me, because he knew an awful lot about cricket!

Stoke Brunswick offered Alexander the chance to further his musical studies in the piano and violin as well as the organ, which he had just started, and also gave him the opportunity to sing in the choir, which the following year gave a medal-winning performance at the International Festival in Rhodes. It was Sue Barber, the school's dynamic Head of Music, who discovered that Alexander had perfect pitch and could sing any note that was called out to him. This led to all sorts of fun and games!

At Stoke Brunswick it was not only his music that shone, but also his football and cricketing skills. In all the teams, Alexander showed tremendous ball skills and co-ordination. Cricket, though, was his main passion and he achieved an extraordinary number of wickets – and on one occasion was triumphantly carried off the games pitch by the whole team. Later, having been talent-spotted at a Tunbridge Wells cricket coaching scheme, he was thrilled to be selected to play for the Kent under-tens. Worried about his physical stamina and faddy eating habits, I used to charge around the Sussex countryside with flasks of high-calorie strawberry milkshake at the ready.

Alexander's health remained fairly stable during the two years that he was at Stoke Brunswick, but now and again, when he became increasingly chesty, he needed the usual two-week course of intravenous drugs. In order to minimise disruption to his studies and sport, I was shown how to administer these myself. This was a complete breakthrough in his treatment –

though it did mean I did the fifty-mile round trip to his school rather more often than I wanted to!

Our house by now was full of huge yellow hazardous waste containers, boxes of needles, syringes and giving sets, and the overflow went into the garage. Giving home intravenous drugs was incredibly time-consuming as it took more than forty minutes to draw them up, with all the correct calculations. Later, ready-made drugs (which we called 'grenades' on account of their plastic grenade-like form) helped to make life easier.

Furthermore, there were often problems with Alexander's line, which let in the flow of antibiotics. It could become blocked or even fall out, and never seemed to last for more than a week. I used to go back and forth to Pembury Hospital with him to have new lines put in, which often took several attempts and were quite painful as they had to be threaded up his arm. This involved using sharp needles. Alexander was always very brave, but he couldn't help crying out in pain after each failed attempt.

Music helped enormously in distracting him from these distressing procedures, and it helped us too as we witnessed his ordeal. Every evening after school he would give us a performance at the piano, playing his latest compositions or a piece that he was learning. Ever a perfectionist, he demanded our complete attention – and used to get very cross indeed if we left our seats for any reason!

As Christian and Patrick settled into their chorister lives, journeys to both Canterbury and Cambridge for services and concerts became part of our weekly routine. Alexander often came with us and I began to wonder if there was an outside chance that he could follow Patrick to King's. But I was also aware that he was already nine, and might have missed the boat, as choristers are normally selected at seven or eight. Alexander's love of singing was very apparent, though, and as an added bonus I felt that it was doing his lungs a lot of good. However, becoming a full-blown chorister would mean boarding, and I wondered how on earth he, and everyone else around him, would cope with a time-consuming, serious illness.

In the end I decided to write to Stephen Cleobury, the Director of Music at King's College, and was struck by his positive reply, which said that he was always happy to hear any boy who wanted to sing in the choir, and following an audition Alexander was offered a place.

The headmaster of King's College School, Nicholas Robinson, was already familiar with CF as he'd had a friend with the disease, and he offered us a tremendously sympathetic ear. The housemaster, Andrew Snowdon, and a rota of three warm and capable matrons ('Matey' Glavannis, Lingwood and Vero), seemed more than ready to give Alexander a chance, and would, during the next few years, go out of their way to help him fight his illness while he fulfilled his chorister duties.

Shortly before he left home for King's, Alexander was fitted with hearing aids, as it was discovered that he was profoundly deaf to high-pitched sound. This was partly genetic and partly drug-induced. However, he hated the hearing aids and refused point blank to wear them, preferring to get by without.

At King's he was given a little room by the matron's office. As well as putting out his medicines and making up milkshakes and at times administering his intra-venous drugs, the matrons accompanied him to those of his outpatient appointments that I couldn't attend (Cambridge being some two hours' drive away), and liaised with Addenbrookes Hospital, which housed a specialist paediatric CF unit.

During the holidays the matrons also went with him on choir tours – on one occasion, even as far as Australia. They were fantastic.

Two weeks into Alexander's first term at King's he had a serious setback in that he became very unwell, with a high temperature and chest infection. I remember driving up to Cambridge late in the evening, lifting him out of bed, and seriously wondering if Tim and I had done the right thing in sending him there. But following a spell in hospital, much to our relief he bounced back into school life.

While in hospital, Alexander was given the option of having a portacath. This is a permanent surgical opening in the chest to receive intravenous drugs. This would have the big advantage of making his needle phobia a thing of the past, but also making life a lot easier from a practical point of view. Alexander seemed fairly happy with the idea, and subsequently had the port inserted under general anaesthetic at Addenbrookes.

His love of sport was undiminished, and one of the matrons, a gifted needlewoman, rustled up a protective white vest, complete with a plastic saucer, cleverly inserted into a little pocket, which fitted snugly over his port.

Since the age of two, Alexander had regularly been seen by doctors at the Brompton Hospital in London, where there is a specialist heart and lung centre, and as he grew older it was there that he went for his regular in-patient stays.

We found the Brompton's Rose Ward to be a wonderfully friendly, welcoming place. Babies, toddlers and children filled the beds, often with parents camping beside them – and the noise, especially during the night, could be impressive! The staff were incredibly kind, patient and good-humoured and they all got to know Alexander very well. Cries of 'Hi Alex' came from all quarters, from the domestic staff sweeping around his bed to the catering team doling out his milkshake.

Professor Andrew Bush led Alexander's team of doctors. He particularly appealed to Alexander, as apart from being very nice (and always wearing brightly coloured ties – the sort with frogs or giraffes on them!), his father was the composer Geoffrey Bush, so there was a real musical connection. In fact, Professor Bush was very keen to plan Alexander's care around his musical commitments, and his first question on the ward round was always, 'When's the next concert, Alex?' I think his entourage on the big ward round were always faintly amused by this!

The one item that Alexander really missed while in hospital was a proper piano, but the hospital school lent him a keyboard and he used to entertain the doctors and nurses and also hold carol concerts at Christmas. Sometimes he went down to practise on the hospital chapel piano if there was no one in there, and at other times he walked across the road to St Luke's church and played the organ there. Harrods, however, which was nearby, provided the best pianos, and on occasion he would be seen hammering away at their Bechstein or Yamaha Grand!

At school Alexander seemed to revel in his life as a boarder and chorister, happily reliant on the attentions of all three matrons. At times, though, he would have lots of tummy ache and feel incredibly tired, needing to have frequent periods of rest. Tiredness was always very much part and parcel of his condition. This was not only because his lungs had to work harder than anyone else's, but the result of the distressing side-effects of his medication, including the extremely strong intravenous drugs, which used to give him a very 'loose tummy'. He needed a lot of emotional support, which the matrons always gave him – and me, too.

I used to worry that his frequent coughing fits might disrupt the chapel services, or irritate the other choristers and choral scholars – not to mention the Director of Music! However, Alexander found ways of dealing with this. He made sure that he had done some physiotherapy before the service, and in chapel managed to perform controlled breathing exercises that seemed to suppress his coughs – for the most part at least. I remember one of the matrons telling me how upset he was when he just could not control a particularly irritant spasm and had to walk out of the service. I mentally wept for him when I heard that story, and wished I had been there to offer support.

By now I had resumed my piano-teaching career, at Somerhill in Tonbridge. Often I used to gaze wistfully at my young pupils, thinking how lucky their mothers were to be able to meet them at the end of the day, to sit with them while they did their homework, to eat supper with them, and then put them to bed. I missed all that deeply.

Each week Tim and I travelled up to Cambridge, armed with our usual supplies of beef stew and shepherd's pie. We loved seeing the boys and supported their games matches, concerts, plays and chapel service whenever we could.

Services in King's College became very special to us, and simply going into the chapel and hearing such beautiful music was so uplifting.

When Christian was in his final year as a chorister, his organ tutor, Tom Williamson, suggested that he try for a place at Eton. Tim and I knew very little about the school, but following a tour and interview with its charismatic Head of Music, Ralph Allwood, we became set on sending him there. To our delight, all three boys were fortunate in gaining awards with means-tested bursaries, which meant that when Alexander arrived there at the age of thirteen he had the support of both of his brothers, with Christian, as house captain, keeping an ever-watchful eye over him.

Eton was only too willing to help and a number of very generous measures were taken. Most importantly, the school provided Alexander with a part-time nurse, Lynne Highy, to assist with all his medical needs. Her generous help enabled him to use his time and energy to focus on his work and not on his condition.

Very thoughtfully, Eton also gave him a ground-floor treatment room – in addition to his study/bedroom – which housed a physiotherapy bed, a small television, all his boxes of drugs, and also a sofa-bed, because at times Alexander's treatment would exhaust him so much that he needed to lie down.

By this time he was taking so many pills daily that they filled a dinner plate. Physically he was able to tolerate them, but psychologically I knew he found it difficult as they were a constant and visible reminder of the disease that he would far rather ignore and so, to the consternation of his carers, he would often delay or avoid taking them.

His busy timetable, coupled with all his medication, often meant that he missed dining-room meals, so he was allowed the use of a small kitchen nearby, to prepare additional milkshakes and to heat up home-cooked meals or food bought locally. Furthermore, boxes of his favourite smoky bacon crisps and Twixes were ordered in by the catering staff – to the envy of the other boys in the house!

It was also agreed that Alexander could use a battery-operated scooter for his journeys across the school's vast campus. This was a huge plus as even walking short distances sometimes made him breathless.

All three boys were looked after by the housemaster, Chris Davis, his wife Innes, and a team of loyal staff. It was a warm and welcoming house, with Lizzie and Millie, the Davis's two young children, giving it very much a family feel.

We both felt extremely grateful to the school for giving our sons such wonderful opportunities. However, as a mother, I still had initial concerns about Alexander going there. Years of taking steroids, combined with his ill health, had left him small and vulnerable and I wondered how he would cope with the hustle and bustle of Eton life. We knew that he would want to visit Patrick and Christian in their rooms, but Christian's room was now near the top floor and Patrick's not far below, both boys having moved up a staircase in an annual order of seniority. Would Alexander have enough puff to make it up there? Little did I realise that five years later he too would be roomed in those lofty heights, despite needing to stop after each flight of stairs to catch his breath.

I wondered too how the other boys in the house would react to him. He didn't want anybody to know about his illness and Chris Davis initially respected that decision, until it became increasingly obvious that the other boys could see all was not well with him. Some thought that he might have asthma or something mildly wrong with his lungs. But the boys popping in and out of his room couldn't fail to notice the pots and pills, feed bottles hooked up to a pump, and the large oxygen concentrator by his bed. Furthermore, Tim and I both knew that Alexander would be in and out of hospital, which would not only affect his academic studies and musical engagements, but also might weaken important peer-group bonds. It was different with the boys who'd come up from King's College School, and those he saw regularly in the music schools. I think he felt more relaxed in their company, and prepared to open up to them – although his illness, I'm pretty sure, would not have been a hot topic of conversation.

The teachers at Eton didn't always know what Alexander was going through, but were at all times patient and supportive, helping him catch up with his studies after prolonged spells in hospital. Christian and Patrick were invaluable in helping Alexander adjust to house life, frequently going to see him, and encouraging him to participate in various activities. Thoughtfully, they used to ring me most evenings, which was very reassuring, and Tim and I visited at least once a week – not least for Tim to mend the scooter, and me to bring home-cooked meals. Chapel services, concerts, house events and team games all provided further excuses for us to visit, and that first summer would see us at various different cricket pitches as all three boys were involved in school matches.

Despite our initial concerns, Alexander slotted happily into Eton life, making new friends and taking advantage of every opportunity that came his way. He was extremely busy in the music department, taking lessons on the piano, violin, organ and harpsichord. His first love, though, was singing in the chapel choir and, in the first couple of years, he was lucky enough to tour America, Australia and New Zealand, with me accompanying him as his carer.

Back home at Highland Oast, suppers were charged with the electricity of Eton life, as the boys recounted endless school stories, often extremely funny, much to the frustration of their sister.

However, during the next few years, infections that led to haemoptysis (coughing up blood) and even lung collapse, would threaten to disrupt this dizzy place, bringing with it a reality check about the seriousness and life-limiting nature of CF. Tim and I had no illusions about the unsettled path Alexander might follow during his time at Eton, so although naturally concerned we were not easily fazed by sudden downturns, and were fuelled, I think, by everyone's desire to help Alexander fulfil his potential, and by his own unfailing cheerful spirit, lively sense of humour, and total acceptance of his illness.

At times, however, we would be particularly challenged. Brilliant highs could, without warning, turn into resounding lows. Following a winning performance in the harpsichord competition during his second year at Eton, Alexander had to be rushed to the Chelsea and Westminster Hospital for emergency treatment to his gastrostomy. The device keeping it fixed had dropped out shortly before the competition and we had no idea that the opening to his stomach could slowly close up within just a couple of hours. Now fourteen, Alexander had to be held down while the staff used forceps to prise the hole open. Afterwards he likened it to a stabbing. His cries of pain and the trauma he went through remain with me to this day.

On other occasions a sudden haemorrhage and subsequent infection of his portacath curtailed valuable choir and orchestra rehearsals, much to his frustration, and soon choir tours at Eton became a thing of the past.

Under the weight of such medical traumas, Alexander started to drop behind in his work. Yet again, support was given by the school in the form of a special timetable that greatly reduced the number of academic subjects he studied, thus easing the pressure.

Throughout his time at Eton, the Brompton Hospital was keen to offer as much support as possible, sending physiotherapists, dieticians and a CF specialist liaison nurse, Jackie Francis, down to discuss his treatment with Lynne and teach her various new techniques in physiotherapy and drug administration. I would often go and help, sometimes staying at my mother's nearby, so that I could offer extra support.

Following Alexander between hospital, school and home was exhausting, though. Apart from the fact that he (like most boys that age) usually left everything for me to pack, I had to make countless journeys back and forth in the car and on the train with a huge amount of baggage, medical and otherwise. Tim was at work, and Alexander was not allowed to carry anything heavy – because with weak bones, induced by all the steroids, he was at risk of fractures – so I became a real pack-horse, and have continued to be ever since!

As he approached adolescence, the disparity of Alexander's size in relation to his peer group became ever more apparent, and I really felt for him. I knew it worried him, but he just didn't want to talk about it.

On one occasion, following yet another blue-light emergency admission to hospital, we were given the news he might not survive the treatment. Memories of Alexander repeatedly clutching my hands, as he lay strapped to the monitor, pale and beaded with sweat as he fought to breathe amid a raging fever, remain vivid. A child psychologist was called in afterwards, not only to help Alexander come to terms with this experience, but to get me through this difficult time. But talk of a possible lung transplant became taboo in Alexander's eyes, being far too dark and 'way down the line' to dwell on, and Tim and I could entirely understand that.

During those teenage years the Brompton Hospital adopted a new policy of segregation for CF sufferers, to minimise the risk of cross-infection. Although this was obviously wise, it did mean that friendships suffered, as patients had to keep to their rooms. Even the hospital school had to abide by the rule, by only ever allowing one child with CF in at a time to use its facilities. As parents, we all felt sad, because we welcomed a friendly chat and a chance to compare notes with one another. Now we were not allowed to mingle in our children's rooms and had to meet either in the little kitchen or the relatives' room. However, on a more positive note, the school's new webcam helped to bring learning to the children's bedsides and the laptop became a very useful means of communication.

This new policy of segregation in the hospital inevitably led to all sorts of illicit meetings between fellow CF sufferers, usually at dead of night, because – like Alexander – they never slept.

We were pleased that so many people visited Alexander, and family relatives, including aunts, uncles and their many cousins, were great in keeping Alexander buoyant. He also enjoyed visits from the boys at Eton who were amazed that Alexander had used, in his time, every piece of equipment in his room!

Chris Hughes, Alexander's piano teacher at Eton, was a regular visitor, taking him off to have a lesson in the chapel at St Luke's and preparing him for the many concerts that he faced. And it was with some pride that Alexander received a standing ovation from all his consultants, nurses, physiotherapists, dieticians and many others, after listening to a twenty-minute recital in the hospital coffee shop, on a piano hired for the occasion. It was only because of their wonderful encouragement that he was able to be there at all.

It was during a chance meeting between Ralph Allwood, the Head of Music at Eton, and Stephen Walker, of Walker George Films, that the idea for a film about Alexander came about.

Alexander, I think, saw the film as yet another challenge that served as a distraction from the regular battles that he faces with his illness, while Tim and I felt the film would raise awareness of CF – and at the same time be a tribute to the tireless efforts of all those who have supported Alexander, both at school and in hospital.

The resulting film, *A Boy Called Alex*, followed his daily life as he coped with his illness and pursued the challenge of conducting Bach's *Magnificat*. He was sixteen when he began rehearsals with the Eton choir and orchestra, and the months leading up to the performance would see him severely ill in hospital, yet as determined as ever to leave his hospital bed to fulfil his commitment.

The film really captured Alexander's character and gave a very realistic portrayal of his life, while at the same time showing what can be achieved by someone with such a serious condition.

But in many ways, his life since the showing of the film has been just as momentous, and in the remaining chapters of this book Alexander recounts in his own words the events of the year April 2008 to April 2009.

Looking back, I sometimes wonder whether, as a mother, I've given the rest of the family enough attention (including Tim). Alexander has always been the main focus in our lives: he got the best cuts of meat, the front car seat, and the most presents. I had to leave the other children for long spells during the school holidays, almost without exception, and they had to take on the roles of cook, cleaner and washer-up, which they did without ever complaining. Sometimes our annual Cornish holiday was interrupted by Alexander's illness and we often had to leave the beach and sunshine in search of local hospitals. But the children's radiant love and support for their brother is only an echo of the wonderful embrace that others have so freely given to him and that we see in so many other families that live with CF.

As I write, it is an early summer's evening. Across the orchards, with their fields of ripening fruit, I can see the shadowy figures of the bee-keepers, moving silently among the hives, their ghostly white suits echoing the cowls of the oasts, speckled in the distance.

We are moving on and, as I sit at my desk, high up in the oast roof, I have time to reflect on our twenty years here in this magical place, which has been the treasured haunt of all our children and that saw Alexander's arrival in the world. Time has continued to hang heavy with the weight and fullness of life (and I would still tell Dr Meyer that), but it has only been so because we have been pulled along by a child, now a young adult, who has continually embraced life's challenges because of his passion for living. And, in doing so, he has brought out the best in so many people.

April 2008

I'd rather not be seen as someone with CF

Spring is one of my favourite times. I've been enjoying it over Easter, but now it's back for the start of my final term at school. When I think of it that way, it feels pretty momentous. I've been at Eton for five years – a big chunk of my life so far – and although I'm looking forward to moving on, school has been a good place for me.

On the first day back, Mum drove me up to Windsor from our home in Kent. It takes an hour and a half, and as usual the car was full of my things – all the school stuff, books, uniform, my cricket bag, and the stack of medicines that I have to cart with me everywhere I go. They filled the entire boot and the back seat. I can't travel light, even for a couple of days, which is a pain. And when I'm away for a few weeks, I need a hell of a lot of stuff.

We got to Eton, which is next to Windsor, by lunchtime and unloaded everything. Then we had to lug it up five flights of stairs to my room on the B

Block corridor in Warre House. The first-years have ground-floor rooms, and then you move up a floor every year. It was suggested by the house staff that I should have a room on the ground floor, which would admittedly save a lot of energy, but it goes without saying that I wanted to be with the other fifth-years on the top floor.

Most people have very fixed ideas about what Eton is like. A school for rich toffs? That it's only for the privileged few who can afford it? That it reinforces notions of superiority, rigid class structure and the old boys' network? For me, all of this couldn't be further from the truth. My parents haven't had to pay anything for my place at the school, and I'm not alone – there are dozens of pupils here on scholarships. Yes, of course there are boys from wealthy families, but there are also a good few from very ordinary backgrounds. And everyone is great.

My experience of Eton has been a really happy one. It's a school that offers a huge variety of activities to do and try. Music is my main thing, and there's a fantastic music department. But there is so much more. The buildings are beautiful, the grounds are extensive, and the equipment – whether you're talking about computers, sports, art or music – is amazing. In that sense, we *are* privileged being here, but most of us appreciate that and try to make the most of the opportunities we've been given.

Life here has never been boring; I've made some

really good friends and have had loads of support from staff and boys alike. The teachers – beaks, as they're known here – are invariably encouraging and put in a lot of effort. Inevitably, as in most schools, there are a few you wouldn't want to get on the wrong side of, but most of them give a lot, and if you're prepared to try, they'll back you all the way. In a minute I'll try and stop this whole 'PR thing' about Eton, but honestly I've got so many good things to look back on during my time here – laughs with my friends, some amazing concerts, brilliant cricket (more on that later), and the opportunity to follow the path that I've chosen.

This term, though, I've got the toughest challenge I've had so far – exams. Over the past few years I've had to miss a lot of exams through ill health. I missed my Common Entrance, my GCSEs and my AS levels (apart from music). For each of these exams I've been in hospital, and although some people might think it's great to miss exams, it was actually bloody frustrating. I certainly didn't want anyone to think it was all a stunt for getting out of them. I'm not someone who ducks things, but, having been ill for so many exams, I was afraid it might be starting to look that way.

This time, there's no missing the exams. I've been offered a choral scholarship to King's College in Cambridge and, to take it up, I have to pass music and history A levels at grade A, history AS level, and

English and maths GCSEs. For me, that's quite a lot in one go, and I do feel a bit daunted. But I'm determined to do it. Going up to Cambridge means so much to me. It's what I've wanted for as far back as I can remember, and if I don't pass the exams, then I can't go. Simple as that. So this time, I'm not going to let anything stand in the way – I'll take the exams no matter what.

Why Cambridge? For me it's all about music. When I was nine I went to King's College prep school and sang as a chorister with the King's College Choir. It's a world-famous male voice choir, made up of sixteen or so boys from the prep school, and another fourteen or so students who are studying at King's. The choir is based in the extraordinarily beautiful King's College Chapel, and they sing at evensong six days a week, and on Sunday mornings, most weeks of the year.

I really loved singing with them as a schoolboy, alongside my brother Patrick, who is two years older than me, and we both wanted to go back and sing with them as students. Patrick – known to everyone as Patch or Paddy – made it. He's studying history at King's and is now in his second year there. It's hard work, studying for a degree and singing for two to three hours a day, but he loves it, and I'm sure I will too. That's why the exams matter so much. Cambridge won't let me off the hook because I have CF. I passed the scholarship audition for the choir last autumn, but I have to prove that I'm up to it academically too. I think I am (or hope so at least), but it feels very nerve-wracking – knowing I *have* to get the grades, or spend the rest of my life wishing that I had.

With all this looming ahead, I came back to school this term with a plan to study hard, do my revision, and not let anything get in the way. I haven't always been great at doing that in the past, but I'm determined to be focused now.

We're lucky here in that every boy has his own room, so no need to share. I'm house captain of games this year and I've got the room Patch had in his last year, when he held the same post. Our elder brother Christian – Chris – was captain of games too. Chris was also house captain, but he was far more organised than either Patch or I are.

The school has been amazingly generous, giving me a treatment room on the ground floor and the help of a nurse who comes in to help me out with my physiotherapy and the various drugs I have to take. It's made life much easier for me to manage.

Once we'd lugged my bags up to my room, Mum and I unloaded the boxes of drugs and special feeds and piled them up in the treatment room. There's a ridiculous number – they stack up against the wall several deep. If I had to keep them in my bedroom there just wouldn't be room. When the final box was in, Mum checked through everything, because (well, according to my mum) I'm hopeless and forget something important.

Eventually Mum headed home. It's never too long before I see her again, as she comes up to school a couple of times a week, with top-up supplies of medicines, and also meals and snacks for me. She works incredibly hard and I'm pretty lucky to have her. My life simply wouldn't happen in the way it does without Mum being there to provide the huge amount of support she gives.

I was glad to be back at school – great as home is, I get restless during the holidays, especially when the others are at work or away. Over the Easter holidays Patch was touring with the choir, Chris was at work – he's working for a bank in London now – and Miranda, our older sister who's doing modern languages at Durham, was studying for her finals. Dad works in the City, in reinsurance, and he's away from home from 7 a.m. to 7 or 8 at night. So that left just me and Mum – though the whole family did get together for a meal on Easter Sunday.

While home, I did a fair bit of revision, caught up on my sleep, talked to friends on Facebook, and practised the piano. But after two or three weeks, those things wear a bit thin and I missed seeing people, so it's good to get back and get on with things.

This term is a bit different to the previous ones. There are fewer classes – or divs, as they're known here – and more study periods, or quiet hours. That's both good and bad. Good because I have a couple of mornings a week when I can sleep a bit later, but bad because I have to motivate myself to study, and I'm not always brilliant at doing that. Having said that, this term I will work with the knowledge that a place at Cambridge is at stake – which is pretty much all the motivation I will need!

My day goes something like this: I get up at about 6.45 a.m., have a shower, check my emails, and then trudge downstairs in my dressing gown. All the papers get delivered each morning for the boys who subscribe to them – I don't subscribe to any, but I have a quick look at the sports pages before heading into the treatment room where I sort out what I need with Lynne, the nurse who comes in most mornings.

After treatment is sorted I rush upstairs, get my tails on, rush back downstairs, and scoot off to classes or to the music block if I'm going to revise. I don't eat breakfast; I can't manage food at that time of the day, and in any case I'm not that keen on cereal.

The uniform – white shirt, stiff collar, black tails and trousers – hasn't changed for hundreds of years. It's kind of Eton's signature and I actually quite like it; it's not as uncomfortable as it looks and it's different. And, like everyone else, we revert to jeans and T-shirts in the evenings and at weekends.

My electric scooter sits outside the downstairs entrance, waiting, like an old friend, to take me wherever I need to go. The scooter was Dad's idea. It's brilliant, as it gets me where I need to go really fast, and I just park it outside on a bike rack or propped against a wall. The first one my parents bought for me was nicked, so I had to get another and, thankfully, I've had this one for a while now. Trouble is it's prone to breaking down. Every couple of weeks the battery goes flat or something snaps and I have to phone my poor dad, who usually manages to get here after work and fix it for me, because I'm really stuck without it. That's commitment. The Eton campus is huge; we have ten-minute breaks between lessons because there's often quite a distance from one building to the next, and I'm not up to that amount of walking.

Anyway, now that it's the summer term it's really nice scooting in the early morning, with the sun in my eyes, a slight breeze blowing and the cheering knowledge that however gruelling the revision is, cricket is a possibility in the afternoon.

Throughout an Eton day you meet all kinds of people, from funny to woefully dull, dodgy to the keenest teacher's pet on earth. But although occasionally the stereotype of an arrogant spoilt young man holds true, most of the boys there are just genuinely nice teenagers.

The best thing about Eton for me has been the music. There's a lot of it, and that's been brilliant. I've been able to play the piano and the organ, sing in the chapel choir, and to conduct as much as I have wanted to. Music is a huge part of my life, bigger than anything else. And here I've been able to do that a lot, fitting it round all the other stuff in school life. I'm really grateful for that. There are a lot of things I can't do – my sporting 'dreams' have had to be put on hold – but I can usually manage to play or sing, and that is a huge deal for me.

I've loved music since I was very small. Not just because of the beauty of the sounds, but because it gives me a kind of freedom. When I'm playing a piece of Chopin, or singing with the choir, I'm not the guy with CF, and everything seems a lot simpler. I spend a lot of my life – more than I like to think about – taking drugs or having treatments. I'm hooked up to machines or being poked, prodded and pummelled every day. So to escape from it all into an incredible piece of music is a truly harmonious way of putting the ogre of CF to one side and getting on with normal living.

Of all the things I am glad of in my life – and there are many – music is right up there at the top of the list (along with having an incredible family). I'm not a religious person, despite the fact that I've always sung a lot of sacred music in choirs, but I do believe that music has a vast amount of power over my actions. Throughout my life I have been fortunate enough to sing in exquisite performances of wonderful music, and can honestly advise people never to underestimate the power of live performance. The first time I sang in a complete performance of Fauré's *Requiem*, even as a young chorister I wasn't immune to the overwhelming sense of calm at the close of the work.

I know I can get carried away on this subject. But who hasn't felt the power of music, whatever music you happen to love, when it brings up feelings like loss, grief, tenderness or joy? It's a language we all share.

I was incredibly lucky because Mum played the piano, and she taught all four of us to play when we were very young. I was three when she first sat me in front of the piano and showed me a few notes. I must have found it exciting and fascinating to be able to make those odd sounds by pressing a key with my finger because I couldn't wait to play more.

We're not what one might call a grand family – far from it in fact. We live in a house where we're always tripping over each other's junk, and the kitchen table jostles for space with the piano. But we are definitely quite a musical family. Dad doesn't play an instrument, but he loves music and he comes to listen to us whenever he can. Mum has always been passionate about music and she teaches at a school near home two days a week.

Our great-grandmother on Mum's side was Grace Hawkins, a composer and pianist, who accompanied the world-famous concert singer Dame Clara Butt. So I suppose that's where we got it from. Mum's mother, my grandmother, is also very musical. She married at seventeen and had seven children, but she still found time to be a piano accompanist in a ballet school for much of her working life. She's eighty-two now – she's great. We still play duets together when she comes over, and I always appreciate her subtle advice when I practise the piano. She had a stroke last year, so it's harder for her to get around now, but whenever she can she comes along to watch when I'm performing.

When it comes to the violin, I started off when my brothers and sister had violin lessons, and I used to have a few minutes with the teacher at the end. Mum also started us singing, and then took us along to the local church choir. We loved it, and singing with choirs became a way of life from then on. My two brothers and I all got into choir schools and sang with the choir at Eton. After Eton, Chris went on to study music at Oxford, while Patch is now with the choir in Cambridge. As for Miranda, she joined in every choral production at her school, Benenden.

It's always (well pretty much, aside from the period when I was obsessed with the organ) been the piano I love best. I started composing little tunes when I was seven. I composed quite a lot, but I didn't like notating the music on paper. Luckily I had a pretty good musical memory and I would just remember it instead. My first composition was called 'Dennis the Menace' and is still on a dusty minidisc somewhere at home!

At the moment I have to fit all my piano practice around revision, which is hard because I'd rather be playing than have my head stuck in a book. I have three or four revision classes each day, and in between there are study periods, when I head for the Rackley library in the music department with a stack of books under my arm, to catch up with practice essays.

I try to practise the piano every day, but I have to admit I'm rather prone to mucking about on the Roland digital piano in my room, rather than polishing a Polonaise, which is what my piano teacher would prefer me to be doing. Then I've got to find time to work on my organ playing too, which is difficult because although it is definitely not my 'first' instrument, it is something I really love. The organ I usually practise on is in College Chapel, the larger of Eton's two chapels, so I have to fit in around services, and anyone else who wants to play. It's a pretty impressive organ to play, a beast with a fantastic sound, but there are so many keen organists at Eton that it's a struggle to get time on it.

Proper 'downtime' at Eton is hard to schedule, but without a doubt my favourite and most relaxing time at school is Saturday afternoon. On Saturday mornings we have classes, but in the afternoon most people are out playing cricket, tennis or even rowing. I really like sport – in fact, I love it, especially cricket. My dream when I was ten years old was to become a professional cricketer who doubled as a musician. If I hadn't had CF, perhaps . . . As it is, I'll be a musician who adores cricket, though sadly I can't play much these days. When I was little I was apparently quite good; at seven I was the Kent team's mascot, and at nine I played for the Kent under-tens. That's something I've got on Patch. He's crazy about cricket too, and he's very good, but he's never played in a county team. Ouch!

CF put paid to my cricketing dreams, but I do still manage to bowl in the occasional match. Otherwise I'll go down to the main cricket ground, Upper Club, and watch the First XI, or to Agars, another sports ground, where a dozen teams may be playing on a Saturday.

Everyone who meets me picks up on one thing very quickly. I just can't stop chucking a tennis ball around. Sounds daft, but somehow having a ball in my hand makes me feel better, and it's a great way of occupying myself and getting rid of some of my restless energy. I bowl them against walls, throw them in the air, or just hold them in my pocket. I keep a large supply in my room (same with cricket balls) and just stick one in my pocket whenever I go out. (Yes, I know *most* people keep change in their pockets . . .)

I was pretty happy about becoming captain of games, though I think maybe the only reason I got asked was because I was the only member of Warre House B Block with an interest in cricket. Good stuff. It was so last-minute that our housemaster only asked me the night before they decided positions for our last year.

My brief is not strenuous – all I have to do is get together a team of eight players from the top three years for a gentle match against another house every Tuesday. However, that's not always as easy as it sounds. The senior boys in our house are just not cricketers (and, with a few exceptions, none claim to be), so I sometimes have to chase and chivvy and threaten to get them out on the pitch. Earlier in the year I also had to pick a team of eleven players for a more serious house 'ties' match on Wednesdays, but sadly we were knocked out (not unexpectedly) in the first round.

If Saturday is the sportiest day of the week, Sunday is the busiest musically. We start with choir practice before the morning service in chapel, which means dragging myself out of bed earlier than I'd like. First thing in the morning is probably the worst time for anyone to sing, and me in particular, so if I manage to make a top G (above middle C) I regard that as a result. People wonder how I can sing when my lungs aren't so great. It's never easy; for every practice or rehearsal I have to put in quite a bit of effort to make par with all the others. But it's worth it because I enjoy it so much and get a lot out of it. Also, the choir makes a consistently wonderful sound and it feels good to be part of it. In the last few years I've become more inclined towards conducting, but I do love singing and I think even though it's tough sometimes, it's incredible physiotherapy for my lungs.

We have choir practice five times a week for about fifty minutes each session, but I only manage to make perhaps four of those because occasionally I wake up pretty shattered and in no condition to sing. My voice has a life of its own; I can't always choose what it does. In my second year here, to my amazement (and everyone else's), I won the treble cup for unbroken voices. But I'm pretty sure that was because I put everything I had into it, rather than because I had the best voice.

Another aspect I have to work on quite hard is controlling my coughing. I cough a lot, simply because my lungs are not in great shape. But I try really hard never to cough during a service or a performance. I cough just before – and then try to hang on to it until afterwards, and generally I can do it.

My parents often come up for the service and meet up with Patch and me afterwards. It's always good to see them, but we don't end up with a lot of time together because Patch and I always have things we've got to rush off to – music practice, meetings, matches and so on. Dad usually checks the scooter and Mum brings in fresh supplies of the snacks that keep me going, has a word with Lynne, and then they head off again.

The medical side of my life is the aspect that takes up the most time, but the one that I think about least. For the most part, my treatments are routine, and just have to be got through. It's not that I resent them – though sometimes I do – but more that I just don't bother to give them space in my thoughts. The treatments keep me alive, I know that, so I do appreciate them, but they're not what really matters to me. I do what I have to do, but most of the time I'm thinking about a cricket match I've just seen, or a piece I want to play, or a friend I plan to talk to, or a trip I'd like to make. Anything but what's actually happening to me physically.

It's never easy to go into all the details, because generally I've kept them to myself, and the very few people who need to know. It's not that I'm embarrassed, just that I don't want people to see me as someone who's 'ill'. I don't think most people who know me do – I hope they don't, anyway. I sound as though I've got a bit of a cold most of the time, but hopefully that's all anyone meeting me would notice.

I've always wanted to be the same as everyone else, and I am really grateful that my parents treated me like a normal child. I know they weren't sure at first about sending me off to boarding school, but I wanted to go. I was always keen on getting involved and wanted to be like my brothers and sing, and I'm very glad they let me.

Anyway, behind the scenes, here's what the medical side involves:

As soon as I wake up – which can take me a while – I detach the feed line that pumps high-energy food into me while I sleep. I've got a gastrostomy – a small permanent surgical opening near my navel. I've had it since I was thirteen, just before I came to Eton.

Every night when I go to bed I attach the line to it. The other end of the line is attached to a pump that I switch on before I go to sleep. I get 2,000 calories overnight.

I need the extra nutrition because I don't absorb a lot of nutrients from what I eat and I need 30 per cent more calories than a normal healthy adult. The feed they give me at night comes in a bag and it's delivered to the school once a month.

The gastrostomy doesn't hurt – most of the time, anyway – and I'm used to it being there. The only time I become really aware of it is when I need to eat. I tend to forget to eat, but when the gastrostomy becomes uncomfortable, and moves in and out with my breathing, I'm reminded that I need food. Good work.

As well as the gastrostomy I've got a portacath in my upper left chest. A silicone bubble, called a port, was inserted just under my skin and it's connected by a plastic tube – a catheter – to a vein. Needles can be inserted into the port and it makes it far less painful to have all the medication that I need, especially when I'm on intravenous antibiotics. Before I had it, the medical staff in hospital had a pretty hard time trying to thread lines and insert cannulas into my arm. It wasn't unusual for them to try seven or eight times, making me scream my head off when I was younger, that is. The problem is that veins get worn out after a while, so sometimes, when they couldn't find one in my arm, they had to stick a cannula into my head or my foot. Both Mum and I remember when I was nine and very ill, the doctor made twenty attempts to jab a needle in my vein. It was excruciating. The portacath was put in after that and made things a lot easier.

I always know what's going on in my lungs. When I wake up in the morning, after lying flat for several hours, my chest feels heavy and uncomfortable. It's full of mucus – a bit like the chest of a heavy smoker, so I'm told, but ten times worse. So I start the day by coughing up as much of the gunge as I can. I get pretty worked up by people who smoke. I'd be elated to have healthy lungs, and to think people are just destroying theirs infuriates me.

Three times a day, in the morning, early afternoon and at bedtime, I have to do my physiotherapy exercises to help clear my lungs. I used to have percussive therapy – this is someone tapping and thumping my ribs for ten or fifteen minutes while I lay on my side or my front. Lynne would do it or, if I was at home, Mum. But now my bones, according to the scans, are getting a bit thin so it's not a good idea. I've got osteoporosis as a result of the vast amounts of steroids I've had, and the doctors are worried that with too much tapping my ribs might break. So, last November, they suggested that I try a new form of physiotherapy. I wasn't keen, to be honest – I'd have preferred to stick with what I was used to – but they insisted. The new therapy, sometimes called autogenic drainage, is basically a series of breathing exercises designed to do the same job as the percussive therapy – but without the risk of broken bones.

The other good thing about the autogenic breathing is that I don't need someone else and it isn't restricted to a physiotherapy 'bed'. But I imagine I must look quite strange while I'm going through the various exercises – huffing, puffing and coughing, all on my own! Very occasionally, if my lungs are feeling particularly heavy, I'll ask Lynne to do the percussive therapy, because I like the tried and tested route, but otherwise I do the autogenic breathing. Personally I feel the results aren't quite as immediate as with the percussive therapy, but I've got the hang of it now and it's going OK.

All the forms of physiotherapy help rid my lungs of mucus, but there's always more there, and I have a fair number of coughing fits during the day. I also have an inhaler, like the ones asthma sufferers use, and also one that sprays steroids into my lungs.

Then we come to the pills front. I have to take about seventy a day and I absolutely hate having to swallow them. Up to fifty of them are enzymes, because my body's short on digestive enzymes. Others are vitamins, steroids, minerals, anti-fungals, antibiotics, pills for my liver and some to combat stomach reflux, which I get a lot.

I have to admit that I'm not always brilliantly

reliable at taking my medication. It's not that I find it hard to actually *swallow* pills; it's just incredibly annoying to have to take so many. I always start with good intentions of taking the whole lot, but sometimes I'm in such a rush that I forget, or just can't face it. But I have plenty of people who remind me I have to take them, and Lynne tries to make sure I do. Crazy as it may sound with my condition, I know I do have a bit of a blind spot about all the pills, and I'm afraid I have been known to chuck a few of them in the bin. I'm always telling myself that I must try harder. I know I need them, and Mum gets worried if she finds out I've missed them – especially if I skip more than a day or two at a time. I don't mean to worry her, it's just that it's such a pain having to take them all. I find it sometimes helps to make it into a game and see how many I can get down at once. My record is fifteen – but after that I just stop counting.

Anyway, after all that is over, I get going for the day. Because I don't feel like breakfast I tend to have a special high-calorie strawberry drink, called a Scandishake, mid-morning, along with two packets of Walkers Smoky Bacon crisps. The crisps are a serious addiction of mine. I absolutely love them. I eat several packets a day. But my primary dependence is Twix bars. It's not unusual for me to put away as many as ten or fifteen Twixes in a day. I tend to snack more than sit down to meals, and the crisps and Twixes keep me going. If I get the odd spare half-hour during the day I nip back to the treatment room to have a rest – and nab a few more Twixes and bags of crisps.

May 2008

A man with a plan

The main thing on my mind – exams apart – when I got back to school was the *St Matthew Passion*. It's Bach's finest work – at least, I think so. A momentous and breathtakingly beautiful three-hour long piece for two choirs, two orchestras and several soloists.

My plan is to conduct it, but I'm also aware of just how big an undertaking that is. As well as the musicians, I would need a venue and rehearsal space. It's too large a project to pull off at a school, and in any case there isn't time before I leave, so it would have to be some time after that.

Ralph Allwood, the school's Director of Music, is probably the one person who could help get the 'project' off the drawing board. A fantastic teacher, he's supported me – and all the other musicians – in every possible way throughout our time at the school.

Ralph's philosophy is to let us try whatever we want to try – within reason – and his love of music is catching. He spends most of his life encouraging all of us to believe that anything is possible if we put our minds to it. Ralph also seems to have boundless energy. He directs choirs, music groups, orchestras and productions – in and out of school – and he runs workshops, composes, and has founded several choirs. Yet he always has time if you need a word.

In fact it was Ralph who gave me my first lesson in conducting. After watching him conduct the choir at Eton for about a year, I decided to ask him if he could teach me – in fact, as a somewhat over-confident fourteen-year-old, I think I was pretty sure I could do better! He said 'fine', and told me to come along for a group session. So Chris, a friend, and I went along and Ralph let each of us try to conduct a piece we would sing in choir. I absolutely loved it, and since then I've taken every opportunity to learn the art of conducting.

Every year at Eton a handful of boys in their last year put on their own concerts. They choose the music and approach the musicians they'd like to take part. So I was very pleased when, a year or two back, a couple of boys asked me to conduct in *their* concerts.

Inspired by some of the others I'd been involved with, I wanted to put on my own concert and I chose Bach's *Magnificat*. Sadly, that was never going to happen as I was not in my final year, so I had to hijack one of my friends' concerts in order for it to happen! It's just thirty-five minutes long, but is a powerful and complex piece that is incredibly uplifting. The text is the canticle of Mary, mother of Jesus, as recounted by Luke the Evangelist, and it's divided into twelve sections for orchestra and choir.

I asked Ralph if I could do it, and he tactfully commented that Bach had in fact written less complex pieces for choir and orchestra. However, I was adamant I wanted to do the *Magnificat*, and so he said alright; approach the heads of wind and strings and get their permission, sort out a list of the musicians you want and then come back to me. I already knew exactly who I wanted, and three days later I had it all sorted. Ralph just grinned when I told him and said 'fine'.

It was only a few weeks after this that he told me there was someone he wanted me to meet. It turned out to be a documentary director called Stephen Walker. Ralph had met him on a plane coming back from the States, they'd got chatting, and Ralph had suggested that Stephen might be interested in making a film about my planning, rehearsing and eventually performing the *Magnificat*.

I knew that Ralph wouldn't have suggested this to Stephen unless he liked and trusted him, but I was a bit surprised that anyone might want to film me.

When I met Stephen I liked him a lot. He seemed a very genuine, honest and thoughtful person, and I was confident that he would do the proposed film well. It was going to be for the Channel 4 Cutting Edge series – which I already knew about, and the idea grew on me. Of course it was very nice to be asked, and I thought it might even be quite good fun, but the key thing was that I realised it could do a lot for awareness of CF, and that's something I obviously feel strongly about.

Stephen made it clear that this would not just be a 'sad film about a kid with CF'. He promised it would be optimistic and not sentimental, and I was certainly all for that. I wanted to bring CF into the public eye, but I also wanted to say 'don't let it stop you doing what you want to do'. The way Stephen put it to me was that he wanted to make a film about a guy who has a debilitating disease conducting the Bach *Magnificat*, including everything that happens along the way. In other words, it was to be an uplifting film, about somebody going for it.

Stephen and his wife Sally George run Walker George films and they went and met my parents, who liked them, and agreed with me that the film could be a very positive thing. We saw another film Stephen had directed, called *Young at Heart*, about an elderly choir and thought it was excellent – very touching and warm.

Even so, before they began filming I was slightly wary. I didn't know what it would be like being followed around by a man – even a very nice man – with a camera, plus his assistant. But in fact it was fine.

Stephen did the filming himself and I got on with him really well. He didn't film all the time, and when he did he was as unobtrusive and considerate as possible.

The only part I had reservations about was that he wanted to film me having some of my treatments, in and out of hospital. I hadn't thought a lot about this aspect at the start, and as I'm pretty private when it comes to my treatments, it wasn't easy to allow the camera in. But I realised that to convey the truth about CF I had to be honest, even if that meant showing part, at least, of what goes on 'behind the scenes' in my daily life.

By the time we'd been filming for six months we were good friends and the *Magnificat* was well on track. The performance was set for March 2007, towards the end of the second term in my fourth year, in the Eton chapel, and the whole thing was coming together. Then, as has happened at a lot of key moments in my life, I came down with quite a serious lung infection five weeks before the performance date, just after my seventeenth birthday.

I had been feeling pretty rough for a few days and was hoping it would go away, when I woke up in the night coughing up blood. A few specks are not unusual, but this was a fair bit. Not being one to disturb people in the night if I can help it, I hung on, but by the time Lynne came in the next morning my sheets could have been props in a bad horror film and I was feeling pretty nauseous. She called an ambulance and I was taken to the Wexham Park Hospital near Slough before being transferred by ambulance to the Royal Brompton Hospital – my regular home from home. I'm there at least two or three times a year when my lungs get infected, but it's only reached the point of a haemorrhage like this one a handful of times, and when it does get that bad, I notice a lot of worried faces around me. Mind you, I'm only half aware of them though . . . when I feel that ill, I'm pretty out of it with the amount of drugs I have to take. As the intravenous antibiotics go through, I become very woozy. I was aware that Mum was there, and my consultant, Professor Andy Bush, was popping in a lot. Ralph came, and Stephen, and of course my family, but I spent most of the first week there just sleeping.

I've had some pretty close calls with my health in the past. When I was nine the doctors did a CT scan and told my parents they couldn't say how long my lungs would hold out and to be prepared for the worst. I made it through that scare, and a few others, but when I was sixteen my right lung collapsed and I couldn't breathe, speak or walk. They managed to get it going again, but I was in the Brompton for three and a half weeks, and missed a month of school. At the worst point it was very scary, but I thought, 'Well, I've had a good innings, I've made it to double figures, so whatever comes after this is a bonus.'

I suppose that's how I look at things – I subconsciously try not to get sucked into the grim stuff. I know I'm not in great shape, so what's the point in dwelling on it? I know myself inside out, and I'm tougher than most people realise. Besides, I think it's better to push yourself than to play safe. I don't want to just lie around and be miserable; I've got so much that I want to do.

Once again I was in hospital for over three weeks that time. I usually hope to be out in two. But my lung function had dropped to 27 per cent, and Professor Bush wouldn't let me go until it was back up to 40 per cent, which is where it hovers on a good day.

When I got back to school all I could concentrate on was the *Magnificat* rehearsals. To get everyone mad keen (and they were already pretty keen) I threw myself into it, rounding up the people I needed. The guys in the choir and orchestra were brilliant; they all did their bit. In the end, 500 people came along to the chapel to hear it and it went pretty well.

It's hard to describe what is so compellingly wonderful about conducting. You have to bring all the elements together – the singers and the musicians – and keep the piece flowing, while galvanising people to give of their utmost. You have to win the respect and attention of the musicians, because they must watch your every gesture. And you have to get them to interpret the piece in the way you believe it should be played and sung, at the right tempo, gently or more powerfully, with more or less vibrato, more or less choir, soloists or orchestra at any given stage. You have to keep the essence of the piece, whether that is tender, majestic or stirring, while giving it your own stamp. You're in charge, but it's not a question of ordering people about; it's more a question of leading them to understand and interpret your vision.

When all of this comes together, it gives you the most incredible high. To hear a piece you have loved for a long time, played in the way you imagined it, is so satisfying. I'm not saying there weren't mistakes, because there were, but overall it worked, and by the time the audience was applauding I felt very, very happy. In fact, it was possibly the most fun I'd ever had.

The *Matthew Passion* was the logical next step for me. At one point I did hope to do Handel's coronation anthems in my last year at school, but there just hasn't been enough time or space – and, frankly, people are probably getting fed up with me conducting anyway.

When I first mentioned the *Matthew Passion* to Ralph he laughed and said 'Oh come on, Alex!' But I've now worked on him a bit and I think he is beginning to believe that I could do it. I can be pretty persuasive when I want to. The *Matthew Passion* is three hours long, and you need stamina as well as musical ability. But if Ralph believes I have the ability,

then I'm confident I will find the stamina from somewhere.

As I mentioned at the beginning of this book, after
the film was shown I got loads of emails and letters.
Some of them were from musicians and singers, saying
they would like to be part of the *Matthew Passion* if I
went ahead with it. I think that in itself helped to persuade
Ralph that I should do it. I know it will involve a huge
amount of work for him, and we'll need to raise the
funds to pay professional musicians and also hire a
venue. But I'm so grateful to him for being willing to
give it a go. I know mine will be the easy part – turning
up for rehearsals when the time comes. Ralph has definitely got the toughest job, but he says he has some
ideas and I believe he can do it. It's going to have to
be next year, because it will take that long to raise the
money, find the musicians, and sort out a venue. Anyway,
Ralph has promised 'to get back to me' on it.

While there are many things I like about school,
the food isn't one of them. It's not that it's dreadful
– it's actually alright – but there are a lot of things
I don't like eating. I know I'm a bit of a picky eater.
It's true that I don't find it easy to eat regular meals,
but I think Mum might be exaggerating a touch when
she says I have 'a problem'. I'm not that good on
fruit and vegetables, I'll admit. But the list of things
I do eat is getting longer. When I was very small I
only ever ate spaghetti hoops and fromage frais. Now
I like chicken, spag bol (OK – maybe just the bol),

peanut butter, McDonalds, Burger King, chips, strawberry milkshake, cod and haddock, custard, bananas, carrots and Cornish pasties. And I love meat, especially steak or beef with Yorkshire pud.

In my room I've got a George Forman grill, which means I can cook steaks on that. But my staples are still the Twixes and smoky bacon crisps – I'd be lost without them. Actually, the trips to those violin lessons in East Peckham when I was four marked the beginning of my love affair with smoky bacon crisps – I can't remember exactly how it started, but I know we've been going steady for a good fifteen and a half years now.

For anyone else this would be a terrible diet, I know. But Twixes and crisps are easy to eat and they keep me going. And I can get away with a lot of salt and sugar, simply because the CF means I'm just not absorbing much of it – most of it goes straight through me.

One of the best eating moments of my life was when I was eleven and I was taken out for a meal by my housemaster, while on a choir tour, in Perth, Australia. I had a massive T-bone steak and thought it was pure magic – so now I have one whenever I can. But sadly there's not much chance of that at school, so I get by on my snacks and the meals Mum brings me. Most of the other guys here know I don't eat the same meals as they do, but I make sure I don't make a big thing of it.

Anyway, when I'm thinking about music, food is usually the last thing on my mind. And when I'm giving a performance, I can't face eating at all – something to do with nerves, I suppose, and the need to concentrate.

In the middle of May I was asked to play in the Albert Hall, for the Cathcart Schools Prom. The Cathcart is a really pretty big event in some ways, like a mini-Last Night at the Proms, and I was asked to play because I was to be given the Concerto Award for an up-and-coming young soloist. I was stunned when I was told. It was fantastic to be given the award, but the idea of playing in front of a packed Albert Hall was somewhat daunting, to put it mildly.

I've sung in the Albert Hall, with King's College Choir, when I was a chorister, but then there were lots of us. This time it was to be just *me*. I was asked to play the slow movement from Mozart's Piano Concerto number twenty-one, a well-known piece which I had heard countless times. Even so, I practised a lot. The last thing I wanted was to fluff it in front of 5,500 people – but unfortunately that's exactly what happened. I felt I played badly and was absolute rubbish.

The whole thing was really strange. I travelled down from school by train and got there early, but even so I literally had about ten minutes in which to rehearse, because there were so many others needing rehersal time. There obviously wasn't much time to get used to a new orchestra – the Royal Philharmonic – and it felt as though I'd barely got my bearings before it was 'off you go', out the door, on to the stage.

By the time the whole thing started, the place was packed and I was bloody nervous. Almost my entire family were there: parents, brothers, uncles, aunts, grandma. When my slot was announced I made my way over to the piano. It was parked in an unusual spot, behind the double basses, and it was amplified, which felt really odd. So nothing was quite the way I imagined it would be. Plus it didn't really help that while I was playing there were two large screens behind me, playing clips from *A Boy Called Alex*, and a film about Africa which was the theme of the night. So, all in all, there was quite a bit going on. But I'm not making excuses. I shouldn't have messed up, and I did. My playing was patchy and I made mistakes.

When I got off the stage I was furious with myself and I couldn't help kicking, punching walls and banging my head against things. Not all of it was on purpose; at times I have next to no spatial awareness and when I'm worked into a state I crash into everything. But one of the music teachers from Eton was there and he was a big help. He said that although he agreed I'd played badly, I'd get over it. I appreciated him being so direct. I'd rather be told the truth than have someone try to humour me by saying I was fine when I clearly wasn't.

I wanted to just slink away, but suddenly a whole crowd of little school kids, aged about seven or eight (they were in a choir that was performing later on) came up and asked me for my autograph of all things. I gave it to them, hoping that as they were so young they hadn't noticed just how bad my performance was!

After that there was nothing to do but get over it, so I went out and joined my brothers and watched the rest of the concert. We were very near the stage and next on was an electric string quartet, who I considered the highlight of the evening. Then I went up to see some friends who were in a box. The view from the box was fantastic. By the end of the evening all the people having dinner on the ground floor were getting completely smashed – and everybody had their Union Jack flags out. The atmosphere was brilliant and – apart from my bit – it was a really great evening.

Afterwards I had to face the rest of my family, who were extremely nice to me about my playing. It's good to have people who believe in you no matter what, and who reassure you, even though I'm sure they must have noticed how bad I was.

Sadly, I had to get back to school the minute the concert ended, so I said goodbye to everyone and caught the 12.20 train with Chris, who was going back to Oxford. He was going to sit his finals. He should have done them last year, but a week before they were due to begin he came off his bike and fractured his skull against a brick wall. He gave us all quite a scare, and he had to spend a week in hospital and miss his exams. He was gutted – and he had a hideous headache for weeks. He had a haematoma the size of a tennis ball in his skull, but thankfully it went down on its own and they didn't need to operate. He had a job lined up with a bank and they kindly agreed to take him on anyway. He did all his financial exams with them, then went back for his finals. It must have been awful to go back and do the revision all over again.

On the train, Chris told me that as well as clips of my documentary they had shown live clips of me playing. Apparently I looked a bit of a prat because my bow tie, which was rather large, was turned 90 degrees and was almost vertical! I cringed when he told me. I must have looked a complete idiot. Made a mental note to check it next time.

During half-term, which was a couple of weeks later, I found myself playing at another concert – this time it was the Cystic Fibrosis Trust Breathing Life awards in the Metropolitan Hilton Hotel. They had got in touch to say I'd won the award for Most Outstanding Achievement, which was very generous of them (I'm never sure quite what I've done to deserve these awards).

The Cystic Fibrosis Trust arranged for me, Mum and Dad to stay in the hotel. It was very luxurious and there was a goody bag waiting for me with all kinds of things in it – including pyjamas, a voucher for a watch, and loads of Next vouchers, plus a bottle of champagne. I gave the last one away – I don't drink alcohol. It just wouldn't be a good idea with the CF, and I guess you don't miss what you've never had.

The award ceremony was in the hotel's ballroom and it went pretty well in the end. I was down to play cabaret music, but I ended up playing some Liszt and, although I could have been better, I wasn't as bad as the previous time.

The award was given to me by Phil Tufnell. Now *there's* a man – Middlesex and England cricketer, 42 tests, 20 one-day internationals, 316 first-class matches. I would have liked to talk to him about cricket all night, but as it was I didn't get to do more than say hello, which was a real shame.

June 2008

Exam week tested limits

By the time I got home for half-term I was feeling a bit rough, and it got worse as the week wore on. I caught a cold, and then had a very sore throat. But I didn't let it stop me jumping on a train up to London to see Lily, though. If I let feeling ill get in the way, I'd never do anything.

Lily – I usually call her Lils – is someone I've been seeing quite a bit of over the past couple of months, and she's a pretty special person. At seventeen, she is a year younger than I am, and I met her on a choral course last summer.

Ralph Allwood runs week-long choral courses in the holidays, for 16–20-year-olds, most of whom have been choristers or singing in some way for a while, or want to be musicians. Some of the Eton boys help out with admin and filing, and last summer Ralph invited me to teach on two of the courses – I was very pleased to be asked and I loved it. I taught the students in small groups, helping them to improve their sight reading and teaching them songs. As well as some serious sacred music, we did an arrangement of Lennon and McCartney's 'Honey Pie' and had a lot of fun. I actually listen to non-classical music quite a lot, though mostly I have to listen to music that is pre-twentieth century. Sometimes I hear something in a shop or on the radio and think 'that's not bad', and I do have some stuff on my iPod, but generally for me it's in the background. I've always liked The Beatles, though, because their songs have such good harmonies.

Lils was on one of the courses, but we didn't actually get to know each other then, though I did accompany some of her singing lessons (she claims I didn't concentrate and was reading *Harry Potter*, Book 7, which is of course untrue). We only got chatting properly when she got in touch with me a few months later and asked to interview me for a student magazine. I said fine, we met up, and things kind of took off from there.

Once we did get talking we couldn't stop. We found we had a lot in common – not just a love of music, but we seemed to get on well, without taking life too seriously. After that, I invited her to a couple of concerts, and she invited me to her home in London, which was very close, coincidentally, to the Brompton Hospital. I met Lils's mum Claire, and her fourteen-year-old brother Francis, and I got on with them both pretty well. Because her dad is also called Alex, Lils started calling me 'the boy'. Contrary to some of my friends' teasing, I don't call her 'the girl', but my nickname has kind of stuck, so that Lily's whole family now call me 'the boy'.

Lily is honest, chatty, and far more intelligent than I am – in fact, she's doing her A levels a year early. She's also happens to be incredibly pretty. In fact, I think she's beautiful, although she protests that she's not. Because she's tall and slim – taller than me, which doesn't bother either of us – she always looks stunning, but what I like most about her is that she makes me laugh (though, to be fair, I'm usually laughing at her and she at me).

Every few days I've been going up from school to her house – it's a fairly easy journey by train – and have spent the evening there. At first I was a bit worried whether her family would mind me being around so much, but they seem fine about it.

I would have liked to have gone up to see her again before going back to school, but by the end of half-term week I was definitely not in good shape; my chest was feeling heavier and I was generally more breathless – always the sign that an infection is building up. My parents were worried, and thought I should go into hospital. But it was such awful timing, being the week before my exams, so I told them I felt better than I actually did.

I wasn't being brave, it was pure self-interest – I just couldn't afford to miss the exams because my priority was getting to Cambridge.

Undoubtedly the sensible thing would have been

to go to hospital, but somehow I felt sure that I could manage and would get through. Call it a gut instinct, or perhaps just a strong sense of how far I can push myself, but I've had so many health scares that I know when I can go just a bit further and when I need to accept the inevitable – going into hospital.

In the end, I did agree to go to the hospital to be checked over – though I was still insisting I was OK. They informed me I was 'stably bad' – which, grim as it sounds, basically meant that I wasn't in good shape, but it wasn't getting worse. In the end the doctor upped my antibiotics, and I agreed to take the exams in the school sanatorium, under the watchful eye of the school nurse. I can't say I felt very happy about it, but it was a fair compromise.

Revising in those last few days was a nightmare. I had very little energy and just wanted to sleep. But I tried to keep a book propped up in front of me whenever I could, in the hope that some of the information would filter in.

I got back to school on the Sunday before exam week feeling pretty dire. I was taking a risk, I knew that, and when I coughed up a bit of blood on my first night back, I was a little worried. I woke the next morning with a terrible sore throat, and wondered how on earth I was going to get through the week.

Mum had said, 'Please be careful Alexander, blah, blah, stop and go to hospital if you need to blah, blah . . .' I'm sorry, I do switch off a bit when she leaves me at school and I promise I'll be careful. But – newsflash – I don't want people to worry, least of all my parents, although it's hard to live my life without worrying them. But when she left, I did promise that I would go to the hospital if I got worse.

Exam week was probably the worst week of my life so far. I felt awful, but I just wasn't going to give in. I'm driven, I know I am, and I can't help being that way. People say I push myself too hard and they're probably right, but nothing gives me more satisfaction than being able to say 'I did it'. I just can't be ultra-cautious. Even so, that week really did push me to the limit – the days were bad and the nights were appalling.

I barely slept because I was coughing non-stop, so I felt incredibly tired and found it hard to eat, so I lost a bit of weight, which obviously wasn't good either. Had to drag myself out of bed every morning.

The week started with my AS history on Monday, which I had to take in the sanatorium miles away from the rest of the school – with the invigilator, a box of tissues, two litres of water, and the exam papers. I had to do all three forty-five-minute papers in one go, which I found rather a lot. I was allowed to do them on the computer, which helped. But even though the sanatorium is actually quite nice, it felt stuffy and horrible and by the time I got to the second and third papers I had such a bad headache I had no idea what I was writing. I was pretty sure it was rubbish, but as soon as I left I had no recollection of anything I had done; my brain collapsed, so I went back to my room and slept for a couple of hours before getting up to revise for the next exam.

That night I couldn't get to sleep until 3 a.m., so I was pretty shattered when I got up on Tuesday to take GCSE English language. It wasn't too bad, but I was even more knackered afterwards. I was supposed to be practising for a concert at the end of the week, but I was just too tired. Even worse, the cricket was on and I hardly got to see any of it! I did manage to catch a snippet of the Kent v. Sussex Twenty-Twenty game at Canterbury, which was a good match. I would have loved to have seen more, but couldn't spare the time.

Later that Tuesday Mum arrived, bringing food, and stayed for a bit. She is pretty dedicated; she travels up and down to see me, brings food, organises my medication; talks to the doctors; and sees that I'm OK – and she never, ever complains. I can get impatient and irritable, wanting to do things my own way, but I think, or rather, I hope, that she understands it's just because I hate feeling dependent.

No one knows me as well as Mum does. She knows the state of my health simply by looking at me. I know she worries a lot, even though I tell her not to, but of course all mothers worry. And I guess the thing is, *she* worries so that she can take *my* worry away. I know she would do anything for me, and I ought to thank her more often than I do. The truth is, I couldn't manage my life without her.

An encouraging phone call later from Lils kept my spirits up and on Wednesday I did a history A level paper, followed by the second part of the English language GCSE on Thursday. I wrote a really dodgy tale which I reckoned was either going to get me a good mark or fail me!

Friday was the music A level paper. By the time it ended I was so tried I was practically seeing double. But I was really happy as well because I had made it through the week and done most of my exams. I thought I might have to go straight into hospital at the end of it all, but in fact I didn't. Despite the gruelling week, I hadn't got any worse and I was very, very pleased. I even managed to play in the concert, though I hadn't done enough practice, so I wasn't brilliant.

I was worried, though, about whether I had done well enough in the exams, and was afraid I'd done *really* badly in a couple of them. But the results are still two months away, so there's no point in torturing myself with it.

I had a couple more exams during the following week, but thankfully nothing quite as intense as that first week. My last exam was on 19 June – not a minute too soon. It was music writing and listening, and thankfully I was feeling quite a bit better, so didn't have to take it in the sanatorium. The listening exam was a complete dodge though – I couldn't hear a thing and mostly had to take a pot shot at the answers. Having bad hearing is really annoying at times like this.

No one's exactly sure why my hearing is impaired. I don't hear well in the upper registers, though middle and lower are all right. It seems to be at least partly genetic – Dad has bad hearing and really could do with a hearing aid. But some of the drugs I've had to take haven't helped – the doctors think that certain antibiotics have probably made my hearing problems worse. It's a frustrating thing for a musician, but I cope by listening as carefully as I can, and really paying attention to what's going on.

I was lucky with one of the questions in this particular exam. The music I had to analyse was something I'd played a couple of months ago and I recognised it from the bit I did manage to hear. But the listening part was definitely touch and go. For the written part they moved us to another room, with a different invigilator, who happened to be Ralph Allwood. We were there on time, but he came sauntering in fashionably late. He saw us with papers sitting on our desks and just said, 'Well, off you go, then.' He didn't realise that what we had in front of us was writing paper, and that we were still waiting for the question paper!

When we finally got the question papers, I was a touch surprised to see that the questions were all about Vivaldi. I think probably all the musicians who sat that exam would agree with me that it was the music we had revised for least. I was lucky, though, because I *had* done a bit of revision on Vivaldi and just had to hope it would be enough to get me through (although I knew I'd spent too long on one question).

When I finally got out of the exam room I felt a huge rush of relief. I was just so, so relieved. We all were in fact. And I felt so good about having made it through the term without having to go into hospital.

The next major event was Leavers' Day at Eton, which was just a couple of days after the exams finished. I've watched the previous years – including Patch's and Chris's years – get to Leavers' Day and I've imagined how great it would feel when I finally got there myself, and was on the brink of going out into the world. But the reality is that it's a bitter-sweet time. Great fun, but also a bit sad. It's strange to realise that you're about to say goodbye to somewhere you've been for five years, and to all the friends you've made there.

There's a tradition at the school that you make a card (called a leaver) for anyone – teacher or boy – you want to thank. You can give as many as you want, but it's better if they actually *mean* something so you don't want to give out loads. It was really nice when I received several really thoughtful ones – some from boys I knew well, others from boys in different years.

The night before our final day a whole crowd of us went to the Tiger Garden in Eton High Street for a curry. It had become a tradition for us to go there, but this time it was special, because it was probably the last time we would all be there together as a group. I'm not mad about curry, but I can just about eat it, and anyway the food wasn't the main point – it was about being around mates for the last time, taking the piss out of them, making a few plans for the summer, and promising to stay in touch. It was a great evening with enough good food to keep us going for several hours! It was sad that it was the last time we'd all be together like that, but life goes on, doesn't it?

Leavers' Day itself, 21 June, had an almost unreal feel to it. After staying up far too long the night before, I woke up far too late – at 9.30. This really wasn't good at all, as the head was giving a talk to the leavers at 9.40. I had just ten minutes to throw on my clothes and leg it. No time for any physiotherapy or pills – they had to wait until later.

I got to the main hall just in time to slip into my seat and hear the head give us some sage advice before wishing us luck for the future – pretty standard chat, but still really nice to hear.

After that we had our last chapel service. We sang 'Jerusalem' and the 'Hallelujah chorus', belting them out at top volume. I find it's impossible not to be moved by music like that, especially in such a historic chapel. And after singing at literally hundreds of services, it felt a bit poignant that this would be our last. The only problem was that I sang so loudly that I ruined my voice, which wasn't good because I was due to sing again later in the day at the school concert, to which all the parents were invited.

It was a great concert, though, with some very moving moments. A good friend of mine, Ben Sheen, played the solo in Rachmaninov's famous Second Piano Concerto, which was just mesmerising. I only played a token part, on the bass drum, but it was fun to be involved.

I had to sing one of the school songs, but as I'd completely over-taxed my voice earlier, it wasn't a great performance. I'm normally upset if I don't do well, but this time it didn't matter; the atmosphere was so good that no one minded about the standard of the performances. At the end of the concert, the applause raised the roof – after which I fell into bed, absolutely wiped out.

The following day we had a leavers' lunch for all the boys in Warre House B Block, at which we gave our housemaster presents and thanked him for watching over us for five years. Afterwards Mum and Dad came to my room to help load five years' worth of my junk into the car. There was so much stuff that Mum had to drive one load home, and come back again for me and Dad and the rest of my stuff.

After finally climbing into the car and heading off in the direction of home, I slumped down in the back. I felt worn out physically, wrung out emotionally, but happy. I'd said all my goodbyes and it was a great feeling to be taking the next step forward.

I think I slept for about twelve hours that night as all the exhaustion from keeping going through the term caught up with me. It felt so good to be able to rest, with nothing on the agenda for the day except one of Mum's amazing roasts, with masses of Yorkshire puds. Bliss.

Miranda was at home too, so we had a chance to catch up. She had just finished her finals, after four years studying modern languages. She was about to take off again, for Barcelona, where she was going to do a certificate in teaching English, and then head for Paris where she was going to work in market research for a year. I know she needs to do it, but I'm really going to miss her. She says she'll nip home as often as she can, and that she's closer to home in Paris than she was in Durham – but it still feels as if she'll be a long way off.

Miranda is the kind of big sister anyone would want. She's bright, funny, and sweet-natured too. We email one another all the time when we're in different places, and we have a few choice nicknames for each other. We tease each other mercilessly, but under-neath it all we're incredibly close, and she's always looked out for me.

Chris has also just finished his finals, but he had to go straight back to work. As I mentioned earlier, he got a job with a bank last year, after finishing univer-sity, but they gave him time off to take his finals. But after that it was straight back to the grindstone. He shares a flat in London now, so he just comes home for the odd weekend, or for family get-togethers.

Patch will be around later in the summer, but he's still in Cambridge, because although term has ended, the choir commitments haven't. They're still singing every day and they're about to go on their summer tour in Brazil – lucky man.

When all of us can eventually manage to be at home at the same time, we'll have a big celebration – simply because we'll all be at home! I love it when we're all together, but it happens less and less these days, because we're all so busy.

I owe my family a lot and I'm very lucky to have them. They've pretty much been the rock in my life, always there for me, steady and supportive. And I know it can't have been easy for them at times – especially for Mum and Dad. They've been there for me every minute of the last eighteen and a half years.

Mum's had to fit her life around my needs, and she would probably have gone back to work full time if it hadn't been for me. As it is, she works part time, so that she can come to wherever I am, bringing me food and medicines, taking me to doctor's appointments, and generally making sure I'm managing. Her unwavering commitment never ceases to amaze me.

Mum has always insisted on calling all of us by our full names. We don't mind, though – in fact, I actually quite like it when my parents (but nobody else!) call me 'Alexander'. The rest of the family call me 'Wags'. Don't ask why – I don't know!

Dad is very patient. He never really ticked us all off or lost his temper when we were little, although for some reason he did seem obsessive about us having clean clothes, showers, neat haircuts and polished shoes. He has always been a good listener, and he loves telling stories – but he takes so long when he's telling one over a meal that his food gets cold. We're all getting exasperated and going, 'Look, Dad, your food's still there' – and he's *still* only halfway through the anecdote!

Family meals are important to him; he likes us all to sit down to eat together. He makes a bit of a fuss of an evening meal, with candles and a glass of wine, even if we're just having pizza.

Dad was going to be a quantity surveyor when he was younger and his dream was to build his own house. Then somehow he got caught up in London life, taking a job in the City. He's worked incredibly hard, but he's a million miles from the 'fat cats' and the 'big bonus' City culture – that's not him at all. He's had to work very hard to provide for all of us. Hopefully one day in the not-too-distant future he can ease off, and perhaps even do something that he'd really love to do.

Miranda, Chris and Patch have always been there for me. When we were growing up, my needs so often had to come first. I try not to think about that too much because I feel pretty bad about it. They never seemed jealous or complained, or resented the attention I got. In fact they used to laugh when I got the best cuts of meat at dinner. They still do. An awful lot of family life has had to revolve around me. It's less true now, I think, but when we were kids everything had to fit in with hospital stays, visits and my treatment. We seldom went abroad on holiday. Apart from a couple of trips to France, the furthest we went was Cornwall.

We don't spend a lot of time discussing feelings, we're not that kind of family. But we all know that we'll be there for one another if we muck up or have a problem. We laugh a lot; we kids are always teasing one another and joking. Perhaps that's how we cope with life, especially the harsher aspects.

July 2008

A nervous month

The weather has been awful lately so I've been catching up with back episodes of *Lost*, which i think is really bloody good – mostly for the longing to escape to such an incredible place. I love the amazing scenery, and the plotlines are always so intricate. The only other TV programme I watch is *Neighbours* – a serious addiction of mine due to the quality of the acting on show; it's just completely compulsive. Aside from that, I try to watch some cricket when it's on – but now Sky has all the matches, I seldom get the chance.

It does feel good to have a bit of free time on my hands. In between watching *Neighbours* and catching up with friends on that bane of productivity, Facebook, I've been driving around the beautiful Kent countryside. I passed my driving test last summer – a brilliant moment – and I absolutely love driving. I told a mate to tell Chris I'd failed, and my brother then rang up and talked to me in a serious but sympathetic tone – before I told him I had in fact passed.

When I'm driving along, listening to my favourite music at top volume (i.e. a volume I can hear), I can forget about all the drugs and drips and tubes and physiotherapy and be the same as any other guy my age. Moments like that are when I'm at my happiest. Lately I've been listening to Mendelssohn's *Song Without Words*, and even have the book on my piano. Nineteenth-century piano pieces are almost always full of vitality and joy.

I don't always feel up to driving, but mostly I'm fine, and it's like a lifeline because we live miles from anywhere. With the car I can visit friends or just pop into town for a bit, or simply drive . . .

Yesterday I went out to spend the Next vouchers I got given in May by the Cystic Fibrosis Trust. I bought dozens and dozens of socks, in all kinds of colours, and I can safely say that my sock drawer is now well and truly stocked. I tend to stick my hand in and pull out any two when I'm half-asleep in the mornings, so most days I don't wear matching ones (a regular talking point among people who know me well).

I've been up to see Lils a couple of times too. I leave my car at the station and get the train up, which makes it all very easy. I really enjoy seeing her. We're both people who tend to think we can get away with absolutely anything if we smile in the right way, but it doesn't work on one another, which is possibly a good thing. I know when she's trying to win me over, and I just laugh at her, and she does the same to me. She's always saying 'you're such a loser' – nice, I know – but the face she makes when she says it makes me laugh.

We've got to know one another very well very quickly. We just seem to be able to understand each other. Lils doesn't make any allowances for me being ill, and I like that because I don't want anyone to – least of all people I'm close to.

She's invited me to go to Tuscany with her, along with her mother and brother, for a week in late August. Spending a whole week together at this stage might be a bit much for some people, but we're both fine about it. Having said that, I think Mum is a little worried about how I'll cope, but I've tried to reassure her that I will.

Lils has already been to our house to meet Mum and Dad, and it went really well. She stayed the night and called the area 'The Orchard' because at the back it looks out over the rolling fields of Kent. We sat in the garden, which Mum has made really pretty, over cold drinks and talked about our impending results – not a good topic, but one that is hard to stay away from. Lils is planning a gap year and wants to go and work in Rome; her family lived in Italy for eight years so they all speak Italian. I do wonder sometimes how our relationship will be with me in Cambridge (hopefully) and Lils in Rome. We'll just have to see . . .

Lils has been a great distraction, as has *Neighbours*

and the cricket, but my thoughts keep straying back to exam results. I really have no idea whether I think I did well enough. What if I didn't? I do in fact have a back-up plan, as I've been offered a place at the Royal Academy of Music to study piano. But excellent as the Royal Academy is, my heart is set on Cambridge, so I'm keeping my fingers and toes crossed and hoping I did well enough to get the grades I need.

I've had a few other things to distract me during the waiting, which is good. A few weeks ago I was intrigued when the Director of Music from Yardley Court, the school where Mum teaches, contacted me through Facebook, asking me to adjudicate for their music competition. Apparently Mum didn't even know about it. I appreciated being asked directly, and not through Mum, and I said of course I would do it. I like the idea of supporting and encouraging younger musicians, but because I hadn't done anything like this before, I wasn't sure whether I'd be any good, or would simply end up making a complete fool of myself – but I was very willing to give it a go.

As it turned out, it was a lot of fun. The children at the school are aged seven to thirteen and I had to listen to some of the young musicians playing their instruments and then give them feedback and choose prize winners. Before it all kicked off I played the piano for them. I tried to appear relaxed, so that the kids who were going to perform would relax, because

I know how nerve-wracking standing up in front of an audience can be.

There was a real range of musical ability and achievement, from grade one piano to grade three trumpet to grade six violin. I tried to make useful comments to each of the children, I got everyone to clap the best ones, and I awarded the prizes. By the end I hoped that I'd made the right choices, and that all the children, whether they'd won or not, had enjoyed themselves and felt good about their performances.

It must have gone alright, because when we'd finished the head asked me if I'd be their guest at their Speech Day, two days later. I said I would – then wondered how I was going to sort out a speech in such a short amount of time. It seemed a slightly unnerving prospect, as I was going to have to talk to the pupils, parents, staff and governors – who would all, no doubt, be expecting me to say something worth hearing.

In the end I thought about what I wanted to say, then made a list of bullet points instead of writing out a whole pre-prepared speech. I didn't want to be just reading it out – I wanted it to sound reasonably relaxed, and to be able to look around as I was talking.

When I got up on stage I felt quite nervous, peering out from behind the podium at what seemed a pretty large and very expectant audience. But once I got into my stride, I don't think I was too bad.

I addressed my talk to the children, rather than

the adults. I told them to follow their passion and go for gold. I said they should always strive to achieve their ambitions, to set their sights on what they wanted, and not let anything get in the way. I said that this had always been my way of looking at life. But I also advised them not to be too hot-headed, and to respect their parents and teachers and listen to their advice. I also talked about what it was like being in hospital, and some of the things I wished I had done – like organising my work better. I have always been a bit all or nothing when it comes to studying. I remember being up at 2 a.m. finishing some work, after matron had gone to bed, when I was still at King's prep! I added that this wasn't a good idea, and how it was much better to work steadily and consistently.

It was a pretty serious speech, and I think Mum was surprised that I hadn't been more 'jokey'. But I wanted to make some real points. In the end I really enjoyed it, and afterwards a lot of the pupils – and some of the parents and teachers – came over and told me how much they'd liked it.

The nicest piece of news since the holidays began came from Ralph, who contacted me to say that the *Matthew Passion* project was well underway and that two choirs, an orchestra and the soloists were already on board, not to mention several people who were willing to join a fund-raising committee.

Ralph's starting point was to ask the Rodolfus

Choir if they would take part. The Rodolfus is often referred to as Britain's most exciting young choir. They're a very talented mixed choir, forty-four strong and all under the age of twenty-five, and most of them are choral scholars or music students. The choir was started by Ralph twenty-five years ago and every summer he invites a handful of new members, from the best of the 350 or so young singers who attend the Eton choral courses, to join. I was really pleased they'd agreed to take part, because I know some of them. They're all experienced and talented singers and working with them will be amazing.

The other choir taking part will be the Ripieno, a smaller choir made up of trebles and altos from the Eton Chapel Choir. They will fit perfectly with the Rodolfus and Ralph will be able to prepare them in advance of the rehearsals.

Six soloists have agreed to take part, several of them former members of the Rodolfus choir. There's Tim Robinson, a tenor, Tom Guthrie, a bass, and Sarah Fox, a soprano. Chris Gillett, another former Rodolfus member, is going to be the Evangelist and Michael George will play the Christus. The final soloist is Michael Chance, a counter-tenor whose son is at Eton. I was bowled over that they all said they would like to do it.

We also have an orchestra – the Southbank Sinfonia – Britain's newest orchestra, made up of newly graduated young musicians. I felt so pleased to hear they wanted to do this with me and I'm finally beginning to believe it really is going to happen. I only hope I'll be able to come up to their extremely high musical standards.

A couple of days after my visit to Yardley Court I went back to Ralph's house in Eton, to meet the fund-raising committee. I knew from Ralph that they were a very experienced and knowledgeable group of people, and I felt extremely grateful that they were willing to put in the time and effort to make the concert happen.

The man at the helm is Martin Denny. He runs the Windsor Festival, so he really knows how to make things happen. Then there is Heather Davies, a former tour manager who is going to be chief fund-raiser, and Roderick Watson, who will be treasurer.

We talked over lunch, everyone with their notepads out – except me. Listening to them discuss it made me realise how much planning it takes to organise such an event. We need to raise £25,000 to pay for the whole thing. That's a huge amount of money so I really hope we can do it.

All sorts of ideas were discussed – a website especially for the project is going to be set up and there were a number of different fund-raising suggestions. It all sounded brilliant. And we have a date and a venue – 5 April next year, at the Cadogan Hall in London. It's a wonderful classical music venue and

I'm really excited – and just a bit nervous – at the thought of conducting there.

Musically it won't kick off until the week before when we go into rehearsals. Until then, there's not a lot for me to do, apart from thanking everyone for helping and signing the letters asking for donations. After that I will just keep in touch with what's going on, and get on with my side of things – getting to know the music and planning the performance. In the coming months, I'm hoping to meet one or two experienced conductors, to get their advice.

The *Matthew Passion*, written in 1727, is the story of the death of Christ, based on chapters 26 and 27 of the Gospel of St Matthew and is part of the vast repertoire of music that Johann Sebastian Bach wrote when he was Director of Music at St Thomas Church in Leipzig. As well as Matthew's Gospel, Bach took poetry, written by Christian Friedrich Henrici, and set it to music. Most of the music is his, but some of the tunes in the piece were written by other musicians. Bach took them and harmonised them, using them to great effect by weaving them into the much larger structure. In his day, schoolchildren in Germany knew these tunes, so people hearing the *Matthew Passion* would have recognised them.

It's a passionate, powerful and dramatic work. Ralph and I have different viewpoints about how some bits should be played and it's really interesting exchanging our thoughts on this, but the bottom line is that I've got to feel happy with the interpretation as I'm the one conducting it. It's certainly a big challenge in comparison to the *Magnificat*, but I think – or, rather, hope – I can do it.

I'm pretty familiar with the *Matthew Passion* – I've listened to it many times, and sung in it as a chorister at King's, and I've loved Bach's work since I was very young. And of all Bach's works – and there are so many – the *Matthew Passion* has the greatest intellectual depth, technical brilliance and beauty.

Lately I've been listening to different recordings – I've heard four so far. The most modern is one my aunt gave me for my eighteenth birthday. It's quite pacey and direct. The oldest (from the 1950s) is much more romantic, slow and lush. It's really useful listening to them all, because it helps me work out how I want it to sound – which isn't the same as any of the four recordings I've got.

The *Matthew Passion* has been performed so many times over the years that there are countless recordings available, but, strangely, Bach was largely neglected after his death in 1750. It was Felix Mendelssohn who rediscovered Bach's music during the following century. Mendelssohn was given a copy of the *Matthew Passion* score for his thirteenth birthday, in 1822, by his aunt, and he first conducted it in Berlin, when he was twenty. Mendelssohn venerated Bach, and he later put on the *Matthew Passion* in the church where Bach had been Director of Music – St Thomas in

Leipzig. In 1894, long after Mendelssohn had also died, Bach was moved from his unmarked grave and re-buried in St Thomas's, the church he had loved.

Hearing some of the stories behind the music only enhances it for me. I like thinking about how Bach felt when he wrote it, how Mendelssohn felt when he first discovered it, and how anyone hearing it for the first time would feel.

It was an extraordinary experience for me when I first sang in it, and to conduct it will be a once-in-a-lifetime opportunity. The wonderful thing about conducting is that it gives you the possibility of performing music you love in the way that you believe it should be performed.

There are many highly dramatic choruses and divinely powerful moments in the *Matthew Passion* which are open to the conductor's interpretation. 'Hail King of the Jews', for instance, calls on the chorus to be sarcastic. 'Truly, this was the Son of God' is a powerful message, spoken by a centurion, but taken up by the chorus. Then there is the deeply moving 'Be Near me, Lord, when Dying' which I think might be at its most poignantly beautiful unaccompanied by the orchestra.

Bach rarely said whether he wanted his music to be played loudly or more softly, so this is one of the choices you have to make when conducting the *Matthew Passion*. At every stage I need to decide how it should sound.

When I listen to the different recordings I always have a reaction – at each stage in the piece I find myself thinking, well, I'd like mine to be faster, or slower, more aggressive, softer, with more voices or fewer, more orchestra or less, more majestic and sweeping, or calmer and quieter. Some of the recordings I have are really slow with huge choruses, lots of vibrato and passion. I want mine to be on the faster side, but occasionally I might stray to a more romantic side too. I want to bring out the drama, so that the audience will be drawn into the story and absorbed by it. I think people will only concentrate for all that time if they *feel* something, so I want to reach their emotions. But I know I've still got a long way to go and my ideas change from day to day. I need to listen many more times, to study the score and become completely familiar with it, and then to mark in the score how every passage should be played or sung.

At the moment I'm just listening to it over and over. I have it on loud, because of my hearing. I've tried a hearing aid, but it just doesn't work for me – too fussy and the sound isn't right. I'd rather manage without.

After a few days at home of eating, breathing and dreaming the *Matthew Passion*, it was good for me to put it to one side for a bit to give a lunchtime organ recital at Reading Town Hall. An Eton boy does it every year, and this year it was my turn.

I'm not a brilliant organist – I love it, but there are a lot of people far better than I am. But I was happy to give it my best shot. A far better organist than me, my friend Ben Sheen, came along to be my page turner. He had got into Christ Church, Oxford, as an organ scholar the previous year, so he really knew what he was doing.

Reading Town Hall has a unique organ. You have to kick a wooden plank – *hard* – to make it louder. It really hurts your toes too. And on top of that, I couldn't pull out the stops, so Ben was running around pulling them out as well as turning my pages, and I was sitting there with my foot throbbing. Afterwards people were very nice about it, but I'm pretty sure I didn't play that well. That's me, though – I've hardly ever come away thinking 'I did a great job'. Perfectionists are always conscious of anything that has gone wrong – even if the audience might not have noticed.

After Reading, I went back to Eton to help out with one of the summer choral courses. This year I decided I would only do one week, as doing two last year was pretty tiring. You really do have to work hard during the week. As well as teaching the students in groups, I accompanied several individual singing lessons a day, an hour at a time. After three or four hours of that, plus the group singing, I was very, very tired. I was able to stay in one of the boys' rooms at Eton, which was good, as it meant I didn't have far to go each evening and I was able to nip back there at lunchtime for my pills and to do the autogenic breathing.

I find teaching really satisfying, and I enjoyed discovering that I can do it. I did another Beatles classic, 'Back in the USSR', with them, as well as Erskine Hawkins's 'Tuxedo Junction', made famous by Glenn Miller, in addition to a sacred piece that I love – Purcell's 'Hear my Prayer'. The students were all really keen and hard-working and we produced some good sounds, but it was nice to get home again at the end of the week and rest.

August 2008

A pretty big deal . . .

There are two things on my mind this month: results day, and my trip to Italy with Lils. I'm really looking forward to Italy, but before that I will find out, six days before we go, whether I've made it to Cambridge. Actually, I've got two results' days to get through – the first, and by far the most important, is the A level and AS level results day on the 14th. A week later it's GCSE results' day, so I'll find out whether I got my English and maths. I'm worried . . . and that's an understatement.

It's hard to convey how much it means to me to get my grades and get to King's. I know there are people like me all over the country, waiting anxiously, worrying, making back-up plans and trying not to lose sleep. I guess every one of us feels that our results matter more than anything else. So I try to keep it all in perspective and to remember that I've had more than my fair share of luck so far in life, and if this goes wrong there will be another path. I *do* try to tell myself that, but I'm not sure I believe it – because if I'm honest it feels as though failing really would be the end of the world in some ways.

Mostly I keep all this to myself. My family know how much it means to me, so there's no point in going on about it. I have been keeping busy listening to lots and lots of music, going for drives, and planning the Italy trip. This will be my first holiday abroad since the family went to France in 2001. I've been on choir tours with Eton since then, but not holidays. And this one will also be my first without my family.

So far this summer my health is not doing badly. After the low point during my exams, I picked up pretty well and I've been stable since then. I'm being reasonably sensible, taking my meds, doing my autogenic breathing, and getting lots of rest. I don't want anything to spoil the Italy trip or, even more importantly, the start of my first term at university – *if* I get the grades that is. So the new, sensible Alex is doing all the things he should – well, mostly, anyway.

Mum is a bit worried about the Italy trip, though I've tried to reassure her. She's talked to Lils's mother, who has promised to keep an eye on me. Mum's worried about all kinds of things – the heat, whether I'll take all my pills and shakes, what will happen if I need a hospital. I think I'll be fine.

I was beginning to feel results' day would never actually arrive, and that I'd be in a permanent state of edge-of-my-seat stress – but then suddenly it did.

I woke up early, having barely slept, feeling very, very nervous and thinking 'right, this is it'. I was up by 7 a.m., which is unheard of for me in the holidays. I wasn't sure what to do with myself, so I went for a drive to calm my nerves. As I drove along I tried to think about a concert I'm going to be taking part in next Saturday. My old Head of Music from Stoke Brunswick prep school has asked me to play in a lovely old country house not far from us, and I was happy to accept.

When I got back from my drive, at around 8.30, I plucked up the courage to open my emails. I knew the results were being sent out by the school first thing. Patch and Mum were at home, but I wanted to go and look at the results on my own, in private. I needed a bit of time to adjust if they weren't good. So I took my laptop up to my room, and logged on.

It was an awful moment as I looked, but in the event a reasonably good one. I got an A for music, an A for my AS level history, and a B for the history A level. I was pleased, because I'd been afraid that I'd done a lot worse – but I wasn't euphoric, because Cambridge had wanted me to get an A for the history. The big question was, would they still accept me? The only way to find out was to ring the King's admissions office.

I went downstairs and told Mum and Patch what I'd got. Both were pleased for me – Mum hugged me, and Patch said he was really annoyed that I'd done better than him in the history AS level. No time to feel evil/smug about that one, though – I needed to find out what King's were going to say.

It took me a nerve-jangling half-hour to get through on the phone, but when eventually I did they said there was a letter in the post confirming that I had been accepted – universities had the results a day earlier, so their decisions were already made.

I had got in! The relief was huge, and I felt unbelievably happy and very excited. It felt like a cataclysmic event, the most important of my life so far. Mum said she was delighted, and Patch said no doubt I'd be pissing him off no end for the next twelve months. (Er, the other way round, I think . . .)

I rang Dad, who was at work, and he was really happy for me too. Then I rang Ralph, who was in the middle of teaching on one of the choral courses. He knew my results already; he too said he was delighted for me.

I also rang Lils, who was really happy too, having got two As and two Bs in her A levels. She's hoping to go to university next year, but hasn't applied yet.

Patch and I decided to drive down to Oxford to see some friends who were having a party to celebrate their results – the rest of the day was a bit of a blur, to be honest. It was just one of those amazing days when every few minutes you remember what's happened and feel a fresh rush of happiness. We partied and celebrated, and got home very late at night, exhausted but feeling on top of the world.

The next day I was wiped out, but I managed the concert on the Saturday, which went reasonably well, and then spent Sunday with Lils, talking about Italy. Her family go often, to a villa in Cortona, a little town in the hills above Florence. She says it's the most beautiful place, and having seen photos I believe her, so I can't wait.

Mum spent the next couple of days sorting out all the pills and shakes for my trip, plus an oxygen cylinder in case I need it. I manage without a night feed when I'm away; I take extra shakes instead, which makes things a lot easier. Mum also packed a fair number of Twixes and bags of crisps, though I definitely intend to try some Italian dishes.

I got up early and Mum drove me to Gatwick for a 5.15 a.m. flight – which I was promptly chucked off. Basically we had phoned the airline previously to ask whether it was OK to take a portable oxygen concentrator on the flight, to which they had said yes. However, when I was comfortably settled in my seat, the captain said he had no knowledge of this and asked me to leave the plane. I was pretty fed up, and had to wait nine hours for another flight.

The actual flight was fine, though, and when I arrived in Cortona the villa turned out to be up a small winding road, on a hillside outside the village. It was absolutely beautiful, with breathtaking views stretching across green valleys and blue hills into the distance.

I was given the small guest cottage, which was a little converted garage next to the main house, and it was nice to have my own space, although Lils's family were lovely. Her mum treated me like one of the family, and her brother loves to banter. It's also quite easy to make him laugh, so I do.

On the second day I phoned home and got my GCSE results – more celebrations because I got an A star for English and B for maths. I was pretty pleased with that. I would have had to re-take them if I hadn't got reasonable passes. After that, I felt I could really relax.

We had a really lovely time, just sitting and talking, or driving around. We went on a day trip to Lago Trasimeno, a stunning lake a couple of hours away, where we had lunch and went on a pedalo, minus Freddy Flintoff antics, although the lake had practically dried up in the heat.

Walking up the hill to the house from the town below was quite tiring for me, but I managed it several times.

We had some lovely food, and I even tried pasta al pomodoro, prepared with what everyone at the table assured me was the best tomato sauce in Italy, made by friends of Lils's family. My family like pasta and rice, but I've always refused to go near them, so this was my first plate of pasta and I decided it actually wasn't bad – though I don't think it's going to replace steak at the top of my food list.

It was good for me to be totally responsible for my own health care. I'm going to have to do that at Cambridge so I've got to get used to it. I did forget my pills a few times, but when Lils realised, she insisted I took them. She adopted the role of medication nagger with exasperating dedication, when all I wanted to do was relax and enjoy the beautiful weather. Lils has always known about my CF – she watched the documentary when it first came out – so it's never been a huge issue, but I was surprised by how much she badgered me!

The house had a piano, because Lils's mum wanted Francis to practise, which he did – a fair bit in fact. And I played a bit too, although the only book of music in the house was Mozart Sonatas, so I played a lot of those. Lils's mum said I was like a juke box – she told me what to play and I played it.

Lils and I also listened quite a lot to the Osmonds 'Love me for a reason' because I'm planning to do a transcription of it for a musical gig at Cambridge. We listened to it far too much, really, and it became the joke soundtrack to our week.

During the week Lils and I talked quite a lot, mainly about her legendary taste in music (some songs are an acquired taste she assures me). Most of the week we relaxed by the pool enjoying the views, punctuated by trips to the local gelateria for ice-cream that was better than any I had tasted before.

Although Lils says I'm her best friend and I in turn would admit she's mine, she can be very blunt and to the point. Here's a quote of Lils's that I got from a friend of hers: 'Alex is such a fascinating person, and so, so sweet, and hilarious, you just sort of forget about the rudeness. I suppose when you fall in love with someone it isn't really a matter of choice. And Alex is so romantic, he says these things that make your heart melt. I think one of the reasons he loves me is that to me he isn't Alex the musical prodigy, or Alex the CF sufferer, but Alex the boy.'

On our last night we went for dinner in the village. We talked about me going to Cambridge and her five months in Rome. It will obviously be hard being in a relationship with so much distance between us. I guess we'll find out. Whatever happens, I'm sure we'll always be friends.

I got back from Tuscany on 27 August and headed straight home to catch up with Mum, Dad and Patch. Mum said I'd lost weight – I often do when I'm travelling, because I find it harder to eat – and I was certainly very tired. We were due to go on a family trip to Cornwall in a few days' time, so I wanted to be well for that. I rested a lot but, frustratingly, over the next couple of days my coughing got worse and I started a terrible headache that just wouldn't go. I wasn't sleeping, so I put myself on oxygen at night.

I've always had an oxygen cylinder next to my bed, because sometimes when I'm having trouble with my breathing, it really helps. I use an oxygen mask, because the alternative is nasal cannula, or prongs – an oxygen tube that goes over each ear and round under your nose, with two little prongs that fit up your nostrils and deliver the oxygen. You always see them in medical dramas, but I hate them, they're so uncomfortable. Not that it's easy sleeping with the mask on, but if I can avoid getting really ill it's worth it.

September 2008

Not quitting yet –
I'm due a good innings

I had hoped that I would shake off any infection and be able to enjoy Cornwall with the family, but sadly over the next few days things got a lot worse. I wasn't sleeping and carried on coughing a great deal and felt exhausted – and I also had blurred vision, which I'd never had before. It was very odd and a bit scary.

On the second night of this month I had a spate of coughing – that included coughing up blood – that lasted three hours. It was very painful and I was getting very fed up indeed. I try not to get too annoyed, because it just doesn't help, but last time I coughed up that much blood was seventeen months ago when I had to go into hospital for almost a month, just before the *Magnificat*. And the time before that was when my lung collapsed, in 2006. That time I coughed up blood for three days.

A lung haemorrhage means a major infection. All night I lay in bed thinking 'Bloody hell, I do choose pretty stupid times to get ill' – this time being just before Cambridge. But by dawn my sheets were soaked in blood and I knew it meant hospital. Not good. I went in to tell my parents and Mum drove me to the Brompton. It's a couple of hours' drive from our house and on the journey there I kept the oxygen mask on and the cylinder beside me.

I felt calmer when I got there. I've been going there since I was a baby, so it's as familiar as a second home – though not one I would choose to spend time in unless I had to.

I got settled in my room – CF patients always have their own rooms because of the danger of cross-infection – and they started me immediately on up to twenty syringes a day of intravenous antibiotics. These can be given via the portacath, but they also decided to give me intravenous fluids through a line into my arm, because I was fairly seriously dehydrated. That was the start of a nightmare. They tried to get the needle attached to the fluid line fifteen times in different places on my arms; but my veins are collapsing and just can't take the needles any more. They finally got the line in, but I was left feeling horribly bruised and sore and hating the whole business.

My lung capacity was down to 29 per cent, which is considered worryingly low. If it stayed like that I'd have a 50/50 chance of making it through the next two years. I felt confident it would go back up again, because it always has so far, and once it's back to around 40 per cent they let me leave.

That first night Mum stayed the night on a camp bed in my room. The doctors were a bit worried about me and apparently told her it could go either way, though no one said that to me at the time. To be honest, I was pretty out of things; the antibiotics knock me out and I just sleep.

I knew I was not in good shape. CF is degenerative, and each time I go back into hospital my lungs are a little worse. I'm not under any illusion about it; as well as my battered lungs, my liver is enlarged, my bones are weak, and my digestive system is not good. I know my body is getting gradually weaker, but I'm nowhere near ready to quit yet.

The doctors have talked to me about a lung transplant, but we all agree that will be for a time when things are considerably worse. If a day comes when I can't walk any more, I'll consider that route. Lung transplants are dodgy. Even if a donor lung is found in time, one in five of the people who receive one die within the first year, and almost half die within five years. So it's a really big thing, and as long as I can avoid it I will. I don't need or like to think about it. Nuff said.

Since I was seventeen and moved from the children's ward into the adult one, my consultant has been Professor Margaret Hodson, who is very nice to me considering what a pain I can be! Before that I was with Professor Andrew Bush, who was very wise and very kind. I liked Professor Bush a lot and

I missed him after I left his care. He wrote me two or three really nice, encouraging letters. He always said that I should do whatever I wanted in life. He never tried to hold me back, saying it was far better for people with CF to be feisty and keep proving their doctors wrong.

In hospital I see so many forlorn little faces among the children with CF. I try to show them that it's better if they can manage not to let themselves feel too frightened – to enjoy what you do and do all that you can.

Of course I get frightened too, when I'm lying in bed feeling extremely rough. Occasionally I let myself go into stupidly dark places, when I wonder how long I will be able to keep annoying people, living in this world. The possibility that an infection will not be fought off is always there. Mostly I don't give in to fears about it. I love life too much and I'm a pretty positive thinker. Sometimes, when I feel low, I play music in my head. When I'm listening to beautiful music, I can't think about dying, the dark space in my mind is filled with the power and beauty of music. And once I'm up and busy I focus on whatever I'm doing, and that way I don't give grim thoughts any room. There's just no point in getting depressed; if I do, I've got less chance of getting back on my feet. And I want to get back on my feet, so I'm tough with myself about putting aside fears and focusing on the good stuff. And right now I've got lots of good stuff:

Cambridge, Lils and the *Matthew Passion* to look forward to. I'm so grateful to have music in my life, because it gives me a focus and something to aim for.

By the second day in hospital I was a little better. Very weak, but I'd stopped coughing up blood, so the antibiotics must have started kicking in. I told Mum to go home and go on the trip to Cornwall the next day. She didn't want to go, but in the end I managed to persuade her. The doctors backed me up, telling her not to worry, that I'd be all right, and that I just needed to rest in hospital for a couple of weeks. So Mum went to Cornwall, reluctantly, and I promised to ring all the family as much as I could.

I was so glad she went; she and Dad both needed the break. But it was hard not to feel just a little bit sad about not being able to go myself. We stay with Mum's twin brother Mark and his friend Shelagh, who rent a house down there, and it's fun. I've always enjoyed Cornwall but haven't been for a couple of years, because last year they went when I was teaching on the choral course. But there was no point in them hanging around for me; all I did was sleep, because of the endless antibiotics being pumped into me. When I'm not on such heavy doses I'm generally a light sleeper because I have a restless, active brain and I'm always thinking and planning. Sometimes I lie awake at night and play back bits of Chopin in my head!

Lils came to see me pretty much every day, which was so nice of her and supremely dedicated. People might think it's difficult to have a girlfriend visit you when you're in such a poor state, but I don't feel embarrassed with Lils. Even when I was groggy, we still chatted. I still managed to tease her – and she of course came back at me with some pretty harsh comments – which I thoroughly deserved, I suppose. Otherwise she just filled me in on gossip here and there, and brought me some top grub to get through.

I spoke to Mum and Dad every day and reassured them that I was doing well. I liked to think of them sitting around the table, eating and talking, and going for walks down to the beach as per usual. I hope next year I'll be joining them.

Ralph came from Eton at the weekend, which was really good of him. We talked about the *Matthew Passion* and he told me that several thousand pounds had already been raised. That perked me up a bit, and after that I couldn't wait to get out of hospital and get on with it.

Chris came to see me a few times too. His flat is in Pimlico, which is not far away, so he can nip over after work. A couple of my uncles came as well to take me out, which was nice, and a few cousins popped in. Mum has five brothers, so I have lots of family on that side.

In between visitors I watched loads of sport and cricket on the TV in my room. It has Sky Sports 1 – the only channel (surprise, surprise) that I wanted to watch. People have, at times, accused me of going into hospital simply for the Sky TV, as we don't have it at home. But while I'll admit it's a bonus, I deny the charge absolutely.

It's not just cricket that I'm watching. I'm also passionate about football, especially Manchester U. When I tell people this they take the mick out of me, but I let their comments wash over me. The family legend goes that my sister had a poster of Lee Sharp, a star Man U player from the mid-nineties, in her room and for some reason that started me off. Now I know everything about Man U and I've watched far too many of their games, although I haven't actually been to Old Trafford yet. I've been to Manchester to sing, and I went once to conduct some Mozart at the Royal Northern College of Music, but I hope my next visit will be for a football match.

Crazy as I am about the beautiful game, cricket will always be my first sporting love. At prep school I once got told off for commentating on the match while I was batting. The head told me, in quite stark terms, to shut up. And that's not the only time I've been told to pipe down. I've noticed people can find me quite annoying when I talk endlessly about sport. I guess I talk about it a lot because I can't play as much as I'd like to. That's a real gap in my life – sometimes I'd give anything to be able to take part in the sports I love. As it is, I have to settle for the odd game of darts – I'm quite good and can get a reasonable score if I concentrate – and following every other sport as keenly as I can. Most people get bored watching Lewis Hamilton go round and round the track. I don't, in fact I find the planning and execution of Formula One amazing. The only sport I find boring is lawn bowls. I honestly think they could make better use of the space.

Ten days after going into hospital I was starting to feel a bit better, though I was still on loads of antibiotics. I really hate all the hospital procedures. I had to have blood taken every other day, which hurts. I've had blood taken literally thousands of times and I find it still hurts just as much. They've got to do it, I know that, but sometimes I feel like yelling 'leave me alone'.

Needless to say, I'm used to the Brompton, having been treated there since I was a baby, and I've stayed here on my own since I was five or six. I was in a children's ward then – one CF child was allowed per ward. But from the age of eight or nine I've been in a room on my own. With all the germs buzzing around hospitals they felt it was just too risky for CF kids to mix with others. So I've had to learn to like my own company, and keep myself occupied – and I do. But sometimes it gets boring. Very boring. So occasionally I've had to break the rules. I remember one time, when I was ten, I played hide and seek with my friend Verity on all six floors of the hospital during the early hours of the morning. We were caught eventually, but it was worth it – we'd had so much fun.

The hospital was always really good about keeping us children busy. When I was little they brought in members of the London Symphony Orchestra to play for us and all kinds of artists and actors came. We had music workshops and portrait sessions with people from the National Portrait Gallery and we had a jazz violinist and a clarinettist. I loved all that. But now that I'm an adult there's a lot less entertaining going on. There are compensations, though, and the biggest is that once I'm on the mend I can go outside the hospital for short trips to shop or get something to eat. That makes a huge difference, as I don't feel so confined and am having a say in what I do.

So once I'm able to, I often nip out to Sophie's Steak House, down the road from the hospital. They're really nice in there and if they wonder why I come in on my own all the time, wearing my slippers because I've forgotten to change, they don't say so.

Patch, Mum and Dad got back from Cornwall and they came in together. They obviously had a great time and I was really pleased. They said I looked a lot better, but I still need to rev up a gear. After that, Dad came in every day in his lunch hour, often bringing me a burger for lunch, and Mum came in every day except Tuesday and Thursday, when she's at work.

A couple of weeks in, I was getting very restless, which was good because it meant I was getting better.

I spent a lot of time chucking my tennis ball about, or against a wall, simply to break the monotony. I can't bear sitting around with nothing to do. Thankfully I can have my laptop in hospital and it's been a lifesaver. I can get the internet, so I can keep in touch with friends via email and listen to whatever music I want.

I miss the piano an awful lot when I'm in hospital. Normally I just sit down and muck about on it every day. I think I hold a lot of my emotions in my music. Whether I'm feeling angry, frustrated, or happy, I always play the piano. In hospital I can only imagine that I'm playing, while listening. A poor substitute.

Lots of music is very prescriptive; it tells you what it's about. Then there is music that isn't prescriptive – it has no words or story or background. You can let it take you where you want it to. That's the kind I love. I love piano music with no agenda, so it's open to your interpretation; how *you* see it in your mind.

As a child I used to make up stories to go with the pieces I played, and the reason why I love Chopin so much is because it's perfect for this. Some people call his music depressing, but I think it's poignant and beautiful. I read in a book about Chopin that he told a girl to imagine a scene while she was playing his music, and to go with it. That's what I do. It takes me out of myself, to other worlds.

After three weeks and three days I was much, much better. My lung capacity was up to 40 per cent and the infection had subsided, so I was allowed home – thank goodness. I found it very hard being stuck in hospital for so long.

I did use the time well, though. In the long hours lying in bed I made a big decision: to be far more responsible about my treatment in the future. The day-to-day routine of drugs, physiotherapy and more drugs does wear me down, which is why I try not to think about it most of the time. Developments in the England cricket camp or the state of my music is much more likely to hold my interest. And because of that I've often been accused of burying my head in the sand when it comes to my health. Over the years, I've had a fair bit of flak – and a few stern talks – from doctors and other people around me. In the past all the words of warning bounced straight off me; I never really thought about how crucial they were. I would simply chuck the pills in a bin if I just didn't want to take them.

Now I realise that I can't be that naive any more. If I want to stick around – and I do – then I've got to be seriously responsible about my health. It's not going to be easy; I've got to change my way of looking at things, but I'm sure I can do it.

On that positive note I headed home with Mum and set about making up for lost time – with fifteen Twixes and two cooked meals a day. I'm a bit on the thin side still, so I need to eat, eat, eat. Tucked into steak, mash and peas for lunch and lamb chop with roast potatoes for supper. I was so glad to be home and better, feeling like eating again, and raring to go.

I can't wait to get to Cambridge. Term doesn't start for a few days. Most people go up next Friday, 3 October, but the choral scholars go a couple of days earlier, on Wednesday, the 1st. I'd like to go even sooner, settle in and get to know the place, but they won't let me move into my flat any earlier. So I have to wait – something I'm not very good at, as you will already have gathered.

Another decision – a really sad one – I came to during those last days in hospital was that Lils and I needed to break up. It was really tough, because essentially I didn't want to, but I just didn't think it would work for either of us when we're in different places and hardly likely to see each other. We'll both be meeting new people too – she on her gap year, and me at Cambridge. I talked to her and she was pretty down, she thinks I just want to flirt with other girls. Well yes, in a way, I hope to meet lots of people and that'll be fun. But I don't necessarily want to go out with anyone else, I just felt it wouldn't work when we would be living so far apart. I felt really bad about everything. I really hope we'll stay friends, and keep in touch.

I spent the last day of September packing, which in my case meant chucking everything into bags: clothes, shoes, cricket stuff, books, laptop, tennis balls,

CD player, CDs, kitchen stuff, bedding, towels, food. There's loads of stuff you have to take, and that's before the medical 'mountain'. Mum was a bit more organised, which was just as well because I would definitely have left things out.

It's going to be tough managing on my own in Cambridge. I'll have to be very organised – not my strongest asset. And I'll have to make sure I take my meds, do my therapy, and eat. It's going to be a big change from Eton, where there was a nurse on hand. Even though I found it annoying at times, it was actually reassuring to have someone around. And before that, at prep school, there were the three matrons. They shouted at me from time to time, but I didn't mind, because they were all so lovely.

At Cambridge I need to be responsible for myself. I'm glad Patch is going to be there – for my first year, anyway. It'll probably annoy the hell out of him, but it'll mean a lot to me.

Got to bed very late and lay awake for a while, thinking about life at King's, and how I plan to make the most of it. I can't wait . . .

October 2008

Medication – always a nice topic . . .

Mum and I headed off to Cambridge with the car so loaded down that we could barely squeeze ourselves into it. Piles of bags and cases, plus boxes of tablets, night feeds, all my music, plus five sixteen-bar packs of Twixes. Not to mention dozens of multi-packs of smoky bacon crisps. After all this, there was no room for my scooter, so Mum and Dad promised to bring it up in a couple of days' time. I'd got permission to ride it around college, thank goodness – otherwise my lungs would have been significantly overworked!

A film crew were following us because Walker George are making another documentary to follow up the first one, covering my first few months at university. When Stephen and Sally first asked me, a few weeks back, if they could do a second documentary, I didn't have a problem saying yes. The first had been reasonably fun – I quickly got used to having a camera crew following me around and my friends soon became familiar with it too, and seldom even commented. But I did wonder whether I would be interesting enough to merit a second film.

I talked it over with my parents, as did Stephen and Sally, who seemed convinced that people would like to see me make the transition to Cambridge and follow my efforts to put on the *Matthew Passion*. In the end, as they seemed so sure, and it had worked out well the first time, we agreed to go ahead.

However, this time Stephen isn't directing it himself – he's given it to a director called Paddy Wivell, who seems like a good bloke in general. Paddy and his assistant Maya tagged along behind us on the way to King's. No doubt I'll get to know them well. They've got permission to film in the college, which is good, but it was touch and go – they only got confirmation that they could go ahead the day before we went up to Cambridge.

To make matters worse, I wasn't feeling too great on the drive up; I had a sore throat, cold and cough and my chest was a bit heavy. It's so frustrating when I don't feel completely top-notch for something important. Everyone wants to arrive feeling their best. As it was, Mum didn't want me to go until I was better, but I was keen to go and get stuck into Cambridge life at the same time as everyone else. I would have hated to miss Freshers' Week, when everybody meets everybody, before the academic stuff starts.

I've so often been ill at times that really matter and it's bloody frustrating to be lying in bed when things are going on without me. So I set off for Cambridge hoping that I could pull off the same stunt (doctors' words, not mine) I managed during my A levels and convince myself, and everyone else, that I was fine.

We arrived at lunchtime and the first thing that hit me was the cold. Cambridge is dramatically colder than Kent. They say the Siberian wind blows directly to Cambridge with no mountains in the way to slow it down and I can believe it. The wind cuts through you, and it's only October. But while it was bitter outside, my rooms were boiling because the heating was on full blast. The contrast between inside and outside was – and continues to be – extreme.

I've been given a flat that is set aside by King's College for a disabled student. The advantage is that it is on the ground floor of Bodley's, a block in the main part of King's College. Normally only third-years get into this block – Patch is a couple of floors above me – and it's nice, and very central, but actually I'd rather be with the other first-year choral scholars, who are all in Market Hostel, in town. But I have no choice; the flat is near the porter's lodge and it's got emergency pulleys in it and space for all my meds. Actually I can hardly believe the size of it. Patch's room is much smaller and he even has to go down a few flights of stairs just to have a shower. He's been here working flat out for a couple of weeks, because it's his final year. He came down to say 'hi' and see the flat, and his eyes were out on stalks. I've got a sitting room with a very big desk and a piano – all music students have one – as well as a bedroom, bathroom and a nice little kitchen – now stacked full of cardboard boxes of my shakes, pills and so on.

My desk is facing a beautiful window looking out across a stretch of grass and down to the River Cam, which winds through the town. It's going to be pretty nice sitting at my desk in summer, with all the punts going past. And the living room, bedroom and bathroom all have fireplaces, so it's a very homely place. Patch pointed out that it'll be great for parties.

From where I am, it's less than five minutes (one on the scooter) across the quad to the chapel, which is useful, as I'm going to be spending a fair bit of time there with the choir.

Mum organised my stuff in the flat and then she took off on the long journey back home. I think she'd have liked to stay for a bit longer – I know she was worried about me – but I promised her that I was more than ready to manage on my own.

After Mum had left, Patch came down to help me set up the night feed and we sat and had a chat about the start of term. I think he was happy I'd made it, but it's going to be difficult for him, because he's got a lot on his hands, with finals, the choir, and now keeping me in check too.

That first night I barely slept. I couldn't stop coughing, my throat hurt, and I hadn't got used to sleeping somewhere new. Even so, I woke the next morning thinking, 'This is where I'm going to be for the next three years!' I did feel a little bit anxious too, about whether I can get everything done, in terms of choir and academic commitments and organising my treatment at the same time. I was glad to be sorting it out for myself, but at the same time it did feel a touch daunting.

I spent that first day sorting out books, lecture timetables, supervision dates, and so on. Lectures were due to start a few days later and there would be six or seven a week, mostly in the mornings. Supervisions were mostly in the afternoons or evenings and I would have two or three a week. Everyone goes to lectures, but there are usually only two or three students in a supervision and they last a couple of hours, so no chance to hide in the corner or fall asleep. And we'll have to produce essays and written work that will be scrutinised in great detail. This could be interesting . . .

That first evening I met the other first-year choral scholars for a meal in a local restaurant. One I already know from school, and the others seem like a good bunch. I wasn't feeling on top form, so I wasn't particularly talkative, but I think we all got on.

The first-year choral scholars who I hadn't met before were all great, and two of them (Robbie and Matt) are also reading music. I asked Robbie if he'd be my note-taker if I'm unable to attend lectures due to my health. Even when I'm there I can't always hear. Anyway, Robbie said 'fine' – he seemed happy to help out so I felt really grateful.

That night felt a bit grim, because I couldn't stop coughing. It's a long, long night sometimes, when I'm lying awake. And the feed tube and the oxygen mask – I'm using oxygen every night at the moment – can be uncomfortable; sometimes I wish I could just rip them off. But on the plus side, my throat seemed a bit better the next morning.

We had meetings all day. First we met the Dean and our Director of Studies (known as the DOS), who both welcomed us and told us a bit about what to expect and what is expected of us. (Which sounded like rather a lot. Clearly no slacking off here.)

We also had our first service in the chapel and met the Director of Music, Stephen Cleobury (known as the DOM). I've known Stephen since my time as a boy chorister here, and have always tried to match his perfectionist attitude when it comes to music. There are fifteen choral scholars this year: the six of us in the first year and nine from the second and third years – including Patch, who is the senior beater or head choral scholar. Then there are the sixteen or seventeen choristers aged eight to thirteen, who come across from King's prep school after lessons each day, some of whom I know from when I was a chorister and they were tiny little things.

When the men of the choir perform on their own, their official name is Collegium Regale, but it's known by everyone as Col Reg. The whole choir was founded by King Henry VI to sing the services in the chapel he built for the college. The chapel itself is a stunning building, which still astonishes me when I walk in. We sing a huge range of music, from medieval and Renaissance to contemporary, and as well as singing for the services we'll be doing regular concerts and tours. We'll be singing for evensong five days a week, from 5.30 to 6.15, with a Mass on Thursday evening at the same time. Taking into account that there's an hour's practice beforehand every time, you can be pretty shattered by the end of it all. And there's a Sunday morning service too – so all in all, a lot of singing.

Normally the choral scholars include six basses, four tenors and four counter-tenors. I'm the fifth tenor, which means they could manage without me if they had to, but I hope that won't happen.

Services began that day, but by the following day I couldn't sing and I felt like a dead weight for a large chunk of the afternoon. My throat was too sore, and my energy was pretty low. It was a really disappointing start for me, though I tried not to let it affect my morale too much.

Mum and Dad came to drop off my scooter and came to the service. I saw them afterwards and they said not to worry about not being able to sing, but I still felt angry with myself. Went back to my room and slept for a bit after they'd gone.

Woke up when Patch came to check on me, wondering where I was. Didn't realise I'd slept for so long. Went to have supper in the college hall. King's has the most amazing dining hall, all wood panelled with enormous portraits around the walls and an ornate ceiling several stories high. Very Harry Potter.

Later on Patch came down and set up my night feed for me. That involves tipping five cans of the feed into a plastic container and hooking it up to the pump, so that all I have to do is plug myself in. I used to be lazy and refuse it if I wasn't in the mood, but I'm past all that now and I'm taking it every night.

On our third day we had the matriculation ceremony in which you formally join the university. You have to add your signature to a vast college records book and have a year photo taken. In all the other undergraduate colleges they wear academic gowns for the ceremony, but we don't at King's – a college historically more rebellious than most – so I just wore a suit and tie.

King's is an interesting college. Probably the grandest and most dramatic, architecturally, and also one of the oldest. The chapel, begun in 1446, took almost a hundred years to complete and is the symbol of Cambridge. It's the one sight all the tourists flock to see; there are almost always quite a few outside, and more around the rather imposing neo-Gothic gatehouse, all taking photos. But despite our grand appearance, we're actually among the most laid-back and informal of the colleges. Not to mention the most politically active.

We had to wait for ages in the chapel to sign the book, then we had to wait even longer outside for the year-group photo. It was really cold and not much fun considering my sore throat and everything else. I stuck it out because I really didn't want to miss matriculation and all that that entails. But the cold made my throat worse, so I was feeling pretty rough.

That wasn't the end of it either. In the afternoon the choir members had to do publicity photos in our cassocks – which meant more hanging around in the freezing cold. By now I was feeling pretty dire – even by my standards. By the time we got to choir practice I couldn't sing and I just mimed the words. I hated having to do that, but I just can't get a sound out when my throat is that bad.

After that we had the matriculation dinner – all the first-years in the hall together, all dressed up and enjoying a three-course meal. I couldn't really eat, but it was good to be there and I had warmed up so felt a little better.

In the middle of it Patch came to the hall and beckoned me out, saying, 'Mum's really worried, can you ring her?' It turned out she'd been trying to get hold of me all day, but I was so busy I hadn't checked my phone messages. She could see the day before that I wasn't in a great state.

I rang and persuaded her to let me stay another couple of days and agreed we would decide then. Perhaps not the best move, but I didn't want to leave, especially not right in the middle of the dinner. Went back in, and after the meal all the freshers went to the bar. It was packed and noisy so I couldn't really hear a word, which was annoying because I don't like to ask names twice or look stupid, though more often than not I do. I fell into bed pretty late and very tired. Nevertheless, I did feel so glad to be part of everything that day.

Still didn't really sleep, so by Sunday morning wasn't feeling too good. Went to the morning service, but walking up the aisle I felt extremely breathless and during the service I began to think that I might as well go into hospital and get myself better sooner rather than later.

I carried on, but Mum had phoned the Brompton Hospital to warn them that I might need to be admitted. After the service I headed back to the flat in the pouring rain, in need of the oxygen supply in my room, and I reluctantly realised that I had to be sorted out and that hospital was pretty much the only option. Patch and Livia, his girlfriend, came to my room and packed up my medications and clothes for me. Later, Mum arrived, exasperated that I hadn't gone to hospital earlier. I tried to explain how much I had wanted to stay for Freshers' Week. Basically, the three of them gave me no choice, but I didn't blame them.

I'm supposed to be treated at Papworth Hospital now. When I was at school in Cambridge I went to Addenbrookes, but their CF unit is for children only, so now I have to transfer to the adult unit at Papworth. I haven't been there yet or met the doctors, so I asked Mum to take me to the Brompton. I just don't want to arrive somewhere new when I'm feeling really rough; I'd rather go and meet the team at Papworth for a check-up later and at least get to know the place a bit before I have to be admitted.

With the traffic very heavy on the M11, it took three and a half hours to drive down to the Brompton. Mum was very worried, because I had difficulty breathing and apparently looked really ill. Not the best day so far.

When we got to the Brompton I didn't have the strength to walk and so had to be pushed to the adult CF ward in a wheelchair. A porter took me upstairs to the unit where they listened to my chest, did a chest X-ray, and checked my oxygen levels. Following various tests, they found that the level of oxygen in my blood was pretty low – 86 per cent. That meant I had to have a blood gas test, which involves sticking a really thick needle in my artery – no little pain. And later they had to take blood out of my hand, which hurt a hell of a lot too – that's usually a thing I wouldn't make too much of a fuss about, but because it had been a long and tedious day it had a worse effect than normal.

The doctors were disappointed in me because I chose not to go to Papworth. But, as I've said, I've been going to the Brompton since I was a baby; I know it so well. Plus people can visit me, and it's considerably easier for my parents to get to.

It turned out I was pretty dehydrated, so I had to have two intravenous drips: one for fluids, and the other for steroids. These are litre-sized bags, which they kept up throughout the day. I'd never been on that combination before.

I was so fed up about having to go back into hospital on my fourth day at Cambridge. I knew there was no point in ranting about it, but I was in an awful mood for most of the day. I had only been out of hospital for two weeks and I so badly wanted to be well for the start of the Cambridge term. I'd looked forward to it for months. It felt like it had been right there and then been swiped away from me.

All I could think, lying in bed in my hospital room, was all the fun of Freshers' Week that I was missing. Of all the times to get ill, that was the worst, and as I had drips and lines all over the place, I felt too ill to move. But I promised myself that this time I would really get better and then do everything I could to stay well.

Mum stayed overnight on a camp bed in my hospital room, something that's only allowed in the adult CF ward when someone is seriously ill. It had been a long day for her too, but, as usual, she didn't complain. She's always calm, but it can't be easy for her.

Lying in bed surrounded by machines I thought about everyone else at Cambridge, getting to know one another, singing, working, socialising . . . I wanted to be there. The thing I worried most about was that I might get left behind. But I was too tired to think for long. I just needed to sleep.

Chris came in to see me the next day and he did a really kind Chris-type thing for me by putting my whole timetable into the diary on my phone and computer. He rang up and checked it all and got me organised so that after that I just had to look at what I was supposed to be doing each day. Every lecture, supervision and rehearsal was in there. Chris is a problem solver and I could definitely do with a bit of his organisational skill. He sees what should be done and does it. The rest of us see it, listen to the cricket, and plan to do it later.

Lils hadn't left for Rome yet and she came in to see me. She said that even though we'd split up, she would have felt bad not coming – pretty nice of her. Anyway she's always good company and I was glad to see her. I think she found it hard to see me so ill – so I tried to distract her by mocking her dress sense. Really not the best move, but it did the job. As she left she promised to come every day, which I advised against as I told her I would probably continue to unleash my anti-fashion chat throughout her visits.

Fortunately, that didn't put her off, and I was very glad, because in between visitors it can get very, very dull. When you're on the intravenous antibiotics you've got to stay in one spot – they last for about an hour and leave you feeling groggy and drowsy and not much use.

I had a call from Miranda and it was good to talk to her. She was still in Paris, and seemed to be having a great time. She's promised to come to a concert the choir are doing in Rome in December. At the moment, she's on a four-month probation in her job, but I'm sure she'll be asked to stay. She's doing a second job too, teaching English to two children, so she's quite busy during the day. Fortunately, she emails Chris and Patch and me a lot with updates of her life wherever she is, but of course I'd much prefer her to be here in England.

There was a doctor on our ward who went to Cambridge. To my amusement, he and Chris got into a long conversation about the financial crisis one afternoon when Chris came. It was actually quite educational! Most of the doctors are really good to talk to; they seem to know a lot about sport and music, which can make things a lot easier when they try to have 'serious' chats with you. A lot of them are beginning to realise I'm never good at taking the chats themselves seriously – I'm always laughing for no reason other than to make the conversations less tense. But don't get me wrong, I do think about the content – a lot.

As per usual, the routine in hospital was dull – stuck in my room on my own because of the risk of cross-infection with other patients. I get up, have my drugs, and do my autogenic breathing, with the physiotherapist supervising me to make sure I'm doing it right. Then more drugs at noon, then more physiotherapy in the afternoon. Not very exciting. But at least I have lots of time to listen to music. And once I was feeling a bit better I started work on my first essay, the title of which was 'Compare Beethoven's Fifth Symphony with Schubert's Ninth' – 1,500 to 2,000 words on how both pieces relate to classicism and romanticism. I know the Beethoven pretty well, but I don't know the Schubert at all, so I went online and listened to it a few times – in the end I was actually surprised at how much I liked it. I knew what I wanted to say in the essay, it was just getting it all down on paper that was a bit of a pain.

Resting in hospital, I thought about everything I was missing at Cambridge. I knew I'd have loads to make up, and everyone would have got into all the work properly. Patch emailed occasionally with news and told me not to worry, that I would catch up and get in the swing of things as soon as I got back. But I didn't want to catch up later – I wanted to be there, doing everything at the same time as everyone else. It just felt so strange to be trapped in a hospital room, surrounded by drips and bottles and machines, when the life I wanted to be part of was going on out there.

Dad sometimes popped over from work and we had lunch together. He brought me McDonalds because generally speaking I don't (because I'm quite fussy) eat the hospital food. He told me about the news and the financial world and it was nice to hear about stuff that was nothing to do with being in hospital. And he cracked jokes – terrible ones, which he persisted in telling.

Like Mum, he's always there for me. He's a perfectionist – that's probably where I got it from. When I was little and first started playing the organ I couldn't reach the pedals of the one in our local church. So Dad made an organ bench for me with a red treble clef on the seat. He took three weeks to make it, and it was perfect; smooth and beautiful.

Mum came most days, usually by train, and bringing bag upon bag of food. I realise she and Dad were pretty worried when I first came in. I don't want them to have to worry about me, so I decided (yet again) to make a real effort to look after myself when I get out.

CF is unpredictable and dangerous, I know that, and so do my family. I don't think about it too often, but I know it's not easy for my parents, living with a lot of uncertainty. Mum has strong religious beliefs and is forever saying that this is not the only life we will lead. Next time around, she says, I'll be well and healthy and able to play music and cricket. I wish I had her beliefs, I'd really like to, but I have a pretty dark view of things. I really don't know what's going to happen, but I'm not sure there's anything else after this life. Nothing so far has convinced me that there is.

I used to get pretty scared when I was little. I don't think I've stopped being scared really, deep down. Mum cheers me up, and I like hearing about her beliefs, even though I'm not sure I share them.

After two weeks in hospital my oxygen levels were up, which was a big relief. When I came in I was in a bad way, but now I'm feeling so much better. I can't wait to be allowed out and back to Cambridge.

Chris came in that day after he finished work. I always like seeing him, but he cruelly got me into a debate about whether Gordon Brown should rule the country, knowing full well that he has a much stronger knowledge of the UK economy than I do. He just pitched me in, which was a bit annoying. But it was fun too and I held my own.

Once I'm on the mend, towards the end of a stint in hospital, and I'm allowed out, I try to get out as much as I can. If I go out for too long I get cold, so I have to keep it short. Just before the end of my stay I played the piano for the first time in a while, at a friend's house. I built up my strength to go outside and made my own way there, by taxi. It was great to be able to play again.

And I got confirmation that I am definitely on the

choir trip to Portugal in late November. I am determined to be well for that.

Another bit of good news is that the fund-raising for the *Matthew Passion* is going well. They've set up an Alex Stobbs Matthew Passion website with video links to YouTube clips from the film and an interview I did with Richard Madeley and Judy Finnigan (as in Richard and Judy) as well as loads about the concert and the musicians. A bit embarrassing, but they've raised a few thousand pounds already, and Ralph says it's all pretty promising.

Feeling desperate to get back to everything, but the doctors want me to wait. Took a tennis ball and banged it against a wall a few dozen times, just to relieve the frustration.

Tonight they've put me on a new night feed because they're worried about me being a bit underweight, so now I have to take in even more calories overnight. Beefcake stuff.

Back to Cambridge, at last. After two weeks and three days in hospital it's not a minute too soon and a big relief.

As usual it took several hours to get discharged from hospital – you have to wait around for the docs to sign you off. When we eventually got back, Mum stayed for a bit and cooked me a meal, and the college nurse, Vicky, came to introduce herself. She seems really nice, and has agreed to come in every morning to organise my drugs and check on me. I'm fine with that – I mean, I really wanted to manage everything myself, but I'm actually grateful for a bit of help.

Mum is going to try to organise a carer, through social services, but that might not happen for a while. The hospital has recommended it and it would be really good to have someone who can come in and help with shopping and lifting things and to cover the days when Vicky is off. She's only meant to work three days a week, but she has kindly said that she'll come in every day until we can find a carer.

I got back into the swing of things pretty quickly with a good first day. Vicky arrived before I woke up and put all my pills out for me. Even I was surprised how good I was about taking them all! Then I scooted off to a couple of lectures in the music faculty and then continued working on the essay I started in hospital before having lunch with a couple of the other guys, who seemed pleased to see me back.

In the afternoon I did my autogenic stuff and then bowled along to choir practice, followed by evensong. Singing again felt great and it was good to be giving my lungs a proper workout – hopefully I'll be able to look forward to being well for the rest of term.

A couple of days later and Mum was back to take me to check in at Papworth so that I can be treated there in the future. It's twenty minutes by car from the college, which is convenient. And they have a CF centre there, with eight beds.

It was very strange going to a new hospital. The consultant was nice and everyone there seemed very efficient, but the fact that it was a completely foreign environment for me was an odd experience. The consultant explained that they need to make all their own records, so they would have to do lots of tests. I kind of wish they didn't, but I can see the point in being thorough.

First off was a CT scan of my chest. I haven't had one for three or four years. They had to put a cannula in my arm and give me a dye to make my lungs show up. Putting in the cannula was OK; the bad part was when the dye went in. It felt like my body was on fire. Seriously 'ow'. It only lasted a minute or so, but that was long enough to disorientate me.

After that they did a few more tests. My lung function is better than it's been for a while, so I was really pleased. Mum was a little bit anxious because they said my lung capacity is still not brilliant – at around 30 per cent, it's actually at a level I'd be quite worried about. The doctor said 'your lungs are in pretty bad shape'. Well, I've always known that. I can't see much point in stating the obvious. I'm more interested in improving my lung function over time – and I know the singing is already doing me good.

Got back to King's and said goodbye to Mum before preparing for chapel with my breathing therapy and warm-up exercises. Then I headed over for practice and evensong. After the awful morning, it feels good to be able to get my voice out, and with the bonus of clearing my chest.

In the evening I went to the bar with a bunch of others. I had my usual pint of water and we all got very merry and had a good time.

Arrived back at my rooms at midnight to find that Patch had set up my overnight feed, which was so kind of him. I think he feels he has to otherwise I might forget it – but I am getting better at remembering. He's a good man. We've devised a system with my room key – we leave it for one another in a hiding place round the corner; that way, he can go in and set up when it suits him, without waiting for me to come back.

Mum is still trying to sort out a carer for me. I'm told I definitely need one, and I admit I could do with the help. It would also take a bit of the burden off Patch which is good, but it's not proving easy to get help. Mum's been on the phone for the last couple of days, going between Kent and Cambridge social services, who are both passing the buck and saying the other should pay. The Brompton and Papworth are both involved too, because they have to do reports on me, and then there's my GP in Cambridge, who's trying to help as well. They're all in the loop, but no one seems to want to make a decision or get something done. Poor Mum is being driven mad.

I'm still coughing, but I'm determined to get through the term. I don't want to miss any more. I'm wrapping up warm because it's freezing, and being of modest build I do feel the cold. I've also been eating a lot more because Mum's really worried about my weight. I don't think my weight is too bad, but it could be better. So I'm being really indulgent and have upped my Twix and crisp intake.

Have got through my first full week since coming back and it's gone pretty well. Got to all my lectures, supervisions and choir practices, and even made it to most of them on time!

Vicky's been coming in every morning early to put out my meds – she's so nice and has a terrific no-nonsense approach. On Mondays I have to take an extra tablet and then leave an hour before food, so she puts it on a napkin and draws a circle round it so that I won't miss it.

I'm still not great at taking my tablets. To be honest, they're a regular pain in the neck. I look at them and actually have mixed feelings about taking them at all. But I'm trying to take my health seriously and getting on with it, plus the overnight feed and oxygen. I've had an oxygen concentrator by my bed for a couple of years, but only used it occasionally until this last hospital stay. Now I have it every night, because I know I'll feel slightly better waking up in the morning.

Since this last hospital stay I've been having oxygen in the day occasionally. Specifically I've found it useful to have some just before I go over to chapel – it just helps my preparation for singing. I'm also on higher-strength antibiotics now, which sometimes make me quite drowsy. However, having thought about it, I'm having a reasonably good year in terms of my health. I mean, up to September, things were going well, then everything went a bit pear-shaped. I really don't want to miss any more of the term, so I'm being careful now.

The singing's going well, despite the outrageous behaviour of some third-years. On Wednesday we first-years opened our music books to find that they had stuck in pictures of the *Baywatch* babes and guys, with the heads of our dons and tutors on the bodies of the guys. We were in the middle of singing the *Magnificat* when we turned the page and saw them! Whoever did it had managed to get them in there in between the rehearsal and the actual performance. We couldn't see the music; we had to improvise while trying to prise the pictures off – and we had to struggle not to laugh out loud, which in some cases led to some very red faces.

We've also had the Freshers' concert. Eight people played, all of them studying music. Seven were amazing – I played appallingly and made needless mistakes in a piece I should have known better. I just hadn't had the time to practise properly. I felt extremely annoyed with myself, but enjoyed the rest of the concert immensely as the other musicians are incredibly talented.

November 2008

I strive to be the same as everyone else

I've been back for a few weeks and I've settled into college life pretty well. My day is less structured than it was at school, and that's really enjoyable. On the other hand, the pressure is quite intense; there's a lot I have to do, and to keep up with work I need to be really motivated.

My day begins – on weekdays, anyway – when my alarm goes off at 7. I roll over and re-set it for 7.30, then 8, and I finally get up around 8.30. Sounds lazy, I know, but I've always admitted that I've never been brilliant at getting up. But these days I really do feel groggy in the mornings and it takes me a lot of effort to get going.

I usually have a lecture at 9, so when I'm finally out of bed I don't have a lot of time. I detach my feed line, wash, get dressed, swallow my pills, stuff a couple of Twixes in my pocket, and jump on my scooter. It only takes three or four minutes to get over to the Music Faculty across the river, so I usually make it to the first lecture on time.

If I've got a couple of lectures with an hour or two's gap in between, I tend to stay over at the Faculty. I get worn out if I try to go backwards and forwards too often, so it's easier to wait, and when I'm really tired I sometimes fall asleep between lectures.

This week I've made it to four or five lectures. I skipped a couple, but they're the ones in which I can't hear a thing. Some of the lecturers have quieter voices than others, and there's no point in going if I can't hear anything at all. Recently I had two lectures in which I couldn't hear a word the lecturer said, but, oh well, I'll get there, I suppose. Just as well that Robbie's taking notes . . .

After lectures I come back and have lunch in hall. There's always a roast option, which is great for me. After lunch, if there isn't supervision, I work in the library. There are usually one or two friends there, so we can take a break together.

A couple of days each week I have an afternoon supervision with one of my tutors, and for these we have to produce a piece of work – usually an essay. I'm not an essay person. I enjoy the reading; of course I find it interesting to read about music and what people thought of it. But writing everything I've read and learned into a succinct summary is something I need more practice at. This week I've had to write 2,000 words analysing harmony and counterpoint and

I've also been working on my first essay for twentieth-century music history. I'm still behind on a lot of the work and trying to catch up with what I missed when I was in hospital, so I do feel under quite a bit of pressure.

Some pieces of work are more enjoyable. For supervision this week we were given two bars of an accompaniment to a song, and told to complete the last fifty bars. It's a Schubert song, so rather romantic. I've accompanied a lot of Schubert songs, so I had fun doing it.

I hate it when I mess up. For one supervision I had to write a counterpoint to go against another part and I felt I did really badly. It didn't help that another guy in my supervision group was pretty much note perfect. I'm tough on myself, but only because I want to do the best that I'm capable of, and when I let myself down I give myself a hard time.

At about 2.30, or as soon as I get out of supervision, which sometimes runs later, I go back to my rooms to prepare for choir. I take my pills, do my physiotherapy, and run through the usual vocal warm-up exercises – scales and so on – to get my voice going. I also drink lots of water, which helps. Then I head over to the chapel by 4 p.m., and I'm there till shortly after evensong ends at 6.15. After that it's back to my rooms to change out of the shirt and tie we have to wear under our cassocks in chapel, and into jeans and T-shirt.

Sometimes in the early evening a few of us have a game of cricket along the corridor outside my room, but the porters are always on the lookout so we have to be careful! Because I tend to be tired after choir I don't always last long, but hate to miss cricket if people are up for it, so I'll go along and give some throw downs and then watch the others – though now it's getting so cold that I can't hang around outside for too long. It really is extraordinarily cold in this part of the world.

I don't always go along to dinner in hall. If I've got a lot of work on, I'll put in another few hours of study. I stop and muck around on the piano every now and then, just to give myself a break because I don't find it easy trying to concentrate for hours at a time.

Most evenings, once I've finished work, or run out of steam, I'll get together with friends. As we're together so much of the time anyway and get on so well, I spend a lot of time with the choral scholars in my year, but I do know a lot of other freshers too now, particularly a group of medics who seem to be more sociable than most, which is understandable considering their workload!

Usually I'll go to the bar, make up for not being able to drink by trying to get other people drunk, and when the bar closes we end up hanging out in someone's room. More often than not it's mine; occasionally I feel guilty about having the flat, so I tend to invite people back to it. And anyway, it's very near the bar, so it's convenient for lazy students.

I really enjoy having a bunch of mates sitting around, chatting and laughing into the small hours, but I do get tired. Having said that, it's worth it, because being with my friends means a lot, and although I'm just trying to be sociable, it's more than that. I strive to be the same as everyone else, just another student, swapping banter, gossiping, and winding each other up. I think this aspect of my life is especially important because I so often miss chunks of time when I'm in hospital, knowing everyone is getting on with things without me, and I give myself a hard time about not being part of it all. That's why when I can be in the thick of things, I will always try to make the most of it, so long as I'm feeling up to it.

The downside is that at the end of the evening everyone rolls out of the door, leaving my rooms littered with bottles and glasses. I leave it all and go to bed, then clear it up in the morning. If I'm lucky, Veronica, the sweet lady who cleans, will do some of the washing-up together with Vicky. Veronica is what's known in Cambridge speak as a 'bedder'. It's short for bed-maker, although these days the bedders just empty the bins, put the vacuum round, and make sure you haven't got anything illicit in your room – like candles, drugs, or fifteen people sleeping on the floor. But Veronica is very kind and often does extra things that I'm sure she doesn't really have to do, and that makes my life easier. I always have the ironing board up in the kitchen and usually iron my shirts on a strictly as-needed basis, but the other day I came back to find that Veronica had gone beyond the call of duty and ironed a whole pile of them!

There's still no sign of me getting a carer. Despite Mum's efforts, it all seems to have gone into limbo. The bottom line is that social services won't provide anyone as long as I'm managing without one. And I am managing – I think. Vicky still comes in every morning – usually before I've even woken up – to put out my pills and check on me. Patch sets up the night feed, Veronica helps with chores, and I manage everything else in between. And of course Mum comes up a couple of times a week. She's taken to bringing microwaveable beef dinners, which are my latest addiction.

Sometimes during the day I let people use my rooms for music lessons or practices. The piano's in the living room, which is bigger than most people's rooms, so several people can gather round it fairly easily. And of course I'm in a central location. So when someone asks to borrow it – Patch quite often does – I go to the library to work or the coffee shop for a bit. King's has a great coffee shop with big squashy sofas where I enjoy settling with a book or having a natter with anyone who happens to be there.

I'm really glad to be able to share the use of my rooms, it doesn't feel like a problem at all. But if I could, I'd still prefer to live with the other first-year choral scholars in Market Hostel. Though the size of my place, and the location, is great, I feel a bit cut off there, because I'm a long way from any of my year group. I'd like to be able to pop in and out of friends' rooms, the way most people do, but that's not an option for me at the moment.

My closest friends are the other first-year choral scholars. As well as Robbie, who's wickedly funny, there's Ray (real name Dave), who undoubtedly has the best chat in the choir – probably the best in Cambridge. Of course, he's also a really nice guy and seems to have a knack of getting on with everyone he meets.

Robbie and I manage to spend quite a bit of time together. Mostly because we have the same lectures and supervisions, but we hang out together in the evenings too. We have the same sense of humour, and we've recently started writing little songs, based on various episodes of Cambridge life, or people we've come across while we're sitting in the bar.

If I've missed dinner I sometimes use my little kitchen and make myself a meal. And lately I've been venturing beyond the microwave to actually cooking something – often quite late at night – after I get back from the bar. However, the smoke alarm is proving to be something of a problem. The other night, around midnight, I decided to cook myself two lamb chops on the griddle and the smoke alarm went off. It's really,

really loud and there's no way to turn it off. The alarm triggers a warning in the porters' lodge, so a couple of minutes later a porter arrived who was, thankfully, able to turn it off. It was embarrassing, but nothing compared to what happened a week or so later when I decided to cook roast beef and overdid it a bit. This time when the alarm went off, not only did the porters come, but also a fire engine and two fire fighters. I felt slightly idiotic, but luckily I have the porters' number on speed dial now, so if it happens again I can ring them and say it's just me cooking.

Some of the third-years in my block weren't too pleased, though, as they were studying, or sleeping, and the commotion disturbed them. Had to go and apologise the next day. So I'm having to be a bit more careful; with finals looming, they like peace and quiet. The other night Patch came down after the bar closed and we worked on a concept medley of 'Barbie Girl' and 'Let it Snow' for the college Christmas rag do. We were enjoying ourselves a lot when I got a Facebook message, 'Can you stop . . . I'm in the room above you and I've got an early lecture tomorrow'. We did – and I apologised again. Maybe Aqua's greatest hits at 1 a.m. isn't the best way forward socially.

Nor were the smoke alarm incidents my only encounters with the long-suffering porters. A few days ago I came back from evensong and opened my door to find chaos everywhere. I'm not the tidiest person, but this was more mess than even I can make and I knew it hadn't been that bad when I left: lamps overturned, things all over the floor and – very oddly – a lot of feathers everywhere.

The culprit turned out to be an enormous black bird which had come down one of the chimneys and got trapped in my flat. Not sure what it was – it looked like a crow. It was flying round the bedroom, knocking into things and creating even more chaos.

I went and found a guy who was passing by to help, but we couldn't get it out and he then had to go. Patch then walked past, but when I told him I had a bird in my room he thought I meant a girl, and told me not to worry and that he'd catch up with me later. He eventually came in, but by this point the bird was going crazy, flying round the room, and it managed to trigger one of my alarm cords. Two porters arrived in seconds, but it took them, Patch and me another fifteen minutes to get the bird out through the window. After that, the porters sent a man to block up the fireplace, but he came when I was out and blocked the living room fireplace – and I know the bird came down the bathroom chimney because there were feathers and bird mess absolutely every-where in there.

Patch turned twenty-one a few days ago. Chris came up after work and took me, Patch and Ashley (another choral scholar) out for bangers and mash at the Cambridge Chophouse. Chris and Patch had to drag me out of the student hustings, where I was enjoying listening to the prospective student union officers making their speeches, some of which were noticeably better than others . . .

We had a great evening. The three of us are really close, but we're also very different. For a start they're both much taller than I am – it's odd thinking that if I hadn't had CF, I would probably be over six foot. As it is, I'm quite happy with my height and it's been more of an advantage than you'd think.

Chris is a real big brother to both of us; he's decisive and confident in managing his life and he's very good at getting on with things. Patch is a bit more relaxed, he loves enjoying himself. I used to think he was a bit too relaxed, but now I think I'm more laid back than he is because he's really trying to knuckle down to work for his finals. And these days he worries about me, however much I tell him not to, so he can get quite bossy with me if I'm lax about my treatment.

When I went out to get Patch a present earlier in the day, my bank card snapped in two in the shop. I didn't have any cash on me, but the woman behind the counter said, 'Oh, don't worry, we know you, you're the boy in that film, just come back and pay us tomorrow.' It was nice to be trusted, but also really weird being recognised like that. It's happened to me quite a few times now and I'm still not used to it. When I agreed to do the film it never occurred to me that I might be recognised so much afterwards. People are always nice, but it can be disconcerting. After chapel the other night I was approached by a couple and their son who had seen the film and wanted to say 'hi'. Apparently their little boy has really got into the piano because of watching me, which is great. I felt very chuffed to think I might have influenced a child to want to play the piano. Then they told me he can play backwards – facing away from the piano, with his hands behind his back. I was pretty jealous – I can't do that!

After the film about 700 people added me on Facebook, and someone even set up an Alex Stobbs Facebook fan club – that's a bit embarrassing, though I did notice there were some pretty fit girls in it. I got an entry in Wikipedia too. All a bit strange. And that's on top of all the letters. Some of them were just addressed to 'A Boy Called Alex – Eton'. They were all kind, some just saying they'd enjoyed the film, others talking about music, and others suggesting all kinds of 'cures' for CF. I was touched that people had bothered to sit down and write, and there are some incredibly kind letters I still have at home.

I did want people to become more aware of CF, and I think to some extent the film succeeded. A fair number of people have told me they didn't realise what CF was, or how tough it could be, until they saw the film. I feel very glad when I hear that, but

. . . It's a funny thing, really, because although I want people to know about CF, I actually find it very hard talking about myself and my health. I've always coped by trying not to think about it and I find that a difficult habit to break. Recently one of my friends said 'you'd never guess that you were ill'. That's the nicest thing anyone could say to me. Perhaps that's because I feel that when people know about my condition – some people, anyway – they act differently; they're more cautious around me and they give me understanding, sympathetic looks, which I hate.

I see CF as something I have to manage, like a job that has to be done. I don't feel the need to go on about my condition because it's a very personal thing and I'd rather deal with it when I'm on my own. Only my family have special access, behind the scenes.

Lils once said she thought I was embarrassed by it. She was amazed that some of the guys at Eton never really knew about it, or realised that when I was away from school I was in hospital. It's true that I don't tell people, but I don't think that's because I'm embarrassed – it's just that I don't want to make it the focus. I want to be with people who aren't thinking about me having CF. I think of myself as a normal person who happens to have a condition that needs managing, and that's how I want other people to think of me.

Of course my closest friends know more than other people do. Sometimes one of them will say 'Are you

OK, do you need a rest?' and I'm fine with that. The other day Robbie said, 'You don't really talk much about how you're feeling, do you?' I said, 'I know, I don't talk about it, and I'm not going to start now.' He was fine with that.

I have probably talked to Lils more than anyone else outside my family. We've been emailing and phoning one another a lot lately, and a couple of days ago she came up to see me. She was over on a break from Rome, where she's working in the archive of the library at the British School and living in a little flat near the Vatican. It was really nice seeing her, although I think I might have annoyed her by talking about some new blonde friends I was making in Cambridge. Oh well . . .

Life is hectic here and weekends are when I try to catch up with a bit of rest. Saturdays are good; no lectures or supervisions, so I can have a real lie-in, which I love. But Sunday mornings are tough. All I want to do is sleep, but I have to be in chapel at 9.40 for three hours and then again in the afternoon for evensong. It's hard for me to make a really nice, pure sound, especially in the morning. A huge effort – but worth it. I love the singing at the moment.

I love the chapel too. It's a great place to take a few moments and just be silent. It's full of history, and it's a very spiritual place. Somehow time stands still in there, everything falls away, and you can just be calm. As a child I was overwhelmed with the size and beauty of it – the wonderful symmetry of the chapel and the soaring sound of the sacred music. As I mentioned before, for someone who spends a lot of time in church, I'm not actually very religious. But there's no doubt that a place like the chapel is full of a very special kind of energy.

I love being in the choir, but sometimes I'd like to be in the congregation, so that I could just listen. When I'm singing, I'm usually absorbed by the technicalities of getting what's on the page in front of me right, so there's no time to listen. I want my singing to sound good because I want the choir to sound good. I always want the congregation – or the audience if it's a concert – to have an unblemished performance. And when things are going well, from a technical point of view, then it's a good feeling – the music is wonderful, the atmosphere is uplifting, and there's nowhere I'd rather be.

We do laugh a lot in the choir, too. The Dean is very strict; he frowns if he sees anything is amiss. The other day Patch arrived straight from playing rugby, with no time to change. He did up the collar of his rugby shirt and put on a tie, and then threw his cassock over his entire muddy kit and somehow got away with it. Good work.

The third-years are still trying to wind us up. We have to kneel and sing at one point during the service and today they took out all the kneeling stools, so that we found ourselves kneeling on the floor, our heads peering over the stalls. We had to try to hover in the air – not easy in a kneeling position while singing. Revenge will have to be sought.

We're going to Portugal in a few days, for a concert, and I really want to be on good form for it, but I'm tired and my voice is feeling a bit rough. I've had to mime for three or four minutes in a couple of services this week.

It's just such a pain when I feel ill and tired. I am very focused on what I want to do, which is a lot, but sometimes I just can't get my body to follow through. There are days when I feel quite overwhelmed – I need to practise for the concert, I need to sing, I need to work on an essay, I need to cook myself some supper because it's late and I haven't eaten, but I can't do anything except crawl into bed and sleep.

There are a few things I just can't fit in here – for instance, I'm finding that I don't get much time to read. I don't mean *study*, I do that, but there's no time to read for pleasure. I've always loved reading. I love the escapism of it. When I was nine or ten I liked to read the Famous Five and Secret Seven books; they were cheerful and jolly and the simplest activity was heaven for the children in the stories. They made me feel both lucky and unlucky at the same time – lucky to read them and be in their world, and unlucky that I couldn't do the things these children were doing. Then at Eton I read history books before I went to bed mainly because I enjoy history so much. They were mostly about the Russian Revolution or nine-teenth-century Europe. But anything up to the Second World War is fine, and I always used to read the same books over and over again. I'd find a book I liked and keep re-reading it because it took my mind off everything.

Obviously, what I *do* love doing at the moment is listening to the *Matthew Passion*. The concert is in my thoughts most days. The fund-raising is going well. The team have approached a number of people who want to support us and have given generously. I want to repay their faith by giving them a really memorable concert. I try to do my bit by agreeing to interviews whenever I'm asked, so that I can talk about it and let people know. I've done a couple of interviews recently and there are several papers and a couple of TV stations that want to interview me nearer to the date of the concert.

In the meantime I've got a Cystic Fibrosis Trust concert at the Dorchester Hotel in London coming up. Chris Hughes, who taught me piano when I was at prep school here, is teaching me again and he was rather annoyed when I told him I have to play for twenty minutes at the concert. He was about to have a go at me for leaving it so late to sort out my music, but I told him I'd worked it all out – I plan to play three Chopin pieces and one Liszt. He calmed down after that, and agreed that it was a good choice.

Patch has said he'll come with me to London (basically he wants to enjoy the hotel), and the Cystic Fibrosis Trust has arranged for a taxi to take us there and back. I wouldn't have time to get there by train after evensong, and it would also be pretty tiring; I'm not sure I'd be up to it at the moment.

Even Patch is tired. In fact, I'm getting a bit worried about him because he's working so hard; I think he needs to chill out a bit and relax. He's been working till 2 a.m. most days.

After the Dorchester gig we're straight off to Portugal for the choir concert – travelling there and back in a day, flying from Stansted, and then a few days later I'm playing the organ at the Royal Hospital in Chelsea, home of the Chelsea pensioners. I'm doing the first movement from Elgar's *Sonata*, and I've asked a friend, an organ scholar, to go with me to pull out the stops, and so on.

I know I'm pushing myself. I'm tired and trying to pack a lot in. Mum urges me to slow down a bit and say no to a few more things. But I want to do it all; I really enjoy it. I couldn't bear to be lying around in my room, with life going on all around me and me not being a part of it.

December 2008

A party in a hospital?
Well, it's certainly different . . .

Almost the end of term. It's been incredibly busy, and sometimes I've really had to push myself to keep going. But I've done it and I'm quite proud of that. Now, after the 5th, there are no more lectures or supervisions until next term – thank goodness. We're all exhausted; it's been so full-on.

The Dorchester concert was both good and bad. Good, because Patch and I were chauffeur driven to the Dorchester in a huge limo, given an amazing room for the night, and told we could order what we wanted from room service – T-bone steaks times two. Bad, because I played twenty minutes of rubbish piano and they showed the highlights on Sky. I'm so glad I didn't see it.

We had to get up early the next day for the trip to Portugal. At least the limo was on hand again to get us to Stansted. I slept the whole way on the plane, apart from when I was woken by the terrible Ryanair jingle.

The tour went really well. The Portuguese audience seemed impressed and were considerably less restrained with their applause than a typical English audience. When we finished, it was back on the coach to the airport and I slept all the way home. Got back to my room very, very late and very, very tired, but happy that I'd made it on the trip. Slept in late the next day to try to recover.

The very next week I was back in London, this time in the magnificent chapel of Royal Hospital Chelsea, the venue for a charity concert in aid of Headway, a charity that does so much for people with head injuries. One of the other performers was Rupert Johnston, a former King's chorister who had suffered a severe head injury some years ago. My friend Peter, who's the organ scholar at King's, helped me prepare before the day on the King's organ, after which I came down to London by train and got the tube to Sloane Square, which is close to the Royal Hospital. The concert went as well as it could have, given that it was a very different organ to anything I had played before. The Elgar piece is really beautiful and Simon Over (who was helping with the organ management during the piece) was fantastic and helped make it all work by turning the pages and handling the stops. All the other musicians played well, but I was shattered, and was dying to get back to Cambridge. As it was, I got back at 1.30 a.m.

It was so cold on the way back from the station

on my scooter that I was enormously relieved to get in and get warm. Cooked myself roast beef again. I'm getting fairly good at it now, and quite into late-night meals.

Most of the other students are about to go home, but not those of us in the choir, because December is one of our busiest times. We're off on tour to Italy and Holland in mid-December, before we come back for the Christmas services. I love tours and concerts and all the Christmas music, so I'm just not missing it, but I'm tired and my chest is heavier than usual – and I know I need to pace myself to get through it all.

I've really enjoyed my first term; the only difficult part was having to go to hospital at the start. But since I got back I haven't missed one choir practice. In fact, I've occasionally covered for others who've been off with flu.

I've made some good friends too. I was a bit worried when I got ill that I'd miss out, but the minute I got back they included me and made me feel part of it. I naturally try to be sociable, and that helps, but I also think I've met some really generous and supportive people.

The work's hard and I have trouble getting all of it done. I love the course because it's so varied, but I've got lots of essays to catch up on and I'm going to have to fit them in somehow. I tend to stick my head in the sand when I've got a work backlog – it's a bit like me and taking my meds – I'd rather pretend it wasn't happening. But there are always people – doctors, parents, and now tutors – to nudge me. Perhaps that's a good thing.

A few days ago Mum and I headed over to Papworth for what could be called a regular MOT – in other words, a health check. I was still stable – or, as they put it, 'stably bad' – so I was very pleased. My lung function was up around 40 per cent, which I felt showed that I had proved I could be consistent with my health, manage on my own, and stay well.

The doctors and the nutritionist are still complaining that I'm too thin, though I think my eating has been pretty good. I guess I just need to eat a hell of a lot more, given the amount I'm doing. But it's not always easy to eat when you don't feel particularly hungry. I promised to try, and to be very consistent with night feeds.

I felt in a really good mood after the Papworth visit, because I'm doing so well. Headed off to chapel and got another bit of good news – I was given my first solo. Actually, it wasn't quite a solo – it was me and two others singing in a trio. It came in a Mag and Nunc (Magnificat and Nunc dimittis) by Purcell and it went reasonably well, I think. I was really surprised and pleased to get a part because most of the time I think I won't have the breath to sing a part on my own. Even if it was simply to sing in a service, it felt good to finally get to experience being the lone singer on a part.

For a lot of our time over the past couple of weeks we've been rehearsing for 'Carols from King's', which will be filmed in a few days' time by the BBC, to be aired on Christmas Eve. It's an iconic event and it's interesting being part of it.

To give it its full title, the 'Festival of Nine Lessons and Carols' is a service traditionally held at Christmas in Christian churches all around the world. It tells the story of the birth of Jesus, in nine short readings, interspersed by carols and hymns. The King's version was first held on Christmas Eve in 1918 and broadcast for the first time by the BBC on the radio in 1928. Since then it has been broadcast every year, apart from 1930, although for security reasons the word 'King's' was not mentioned during wartime broadcasts.

These days we pre-record the televised version in early December, and we also do a live broadcast on Christmas Eve, which is heard on the BBC World Service and on Radio 4, and is repeated on Radio 3 – and on many stations around the world – on Christmas Day. With millions of people due to watch us, and listen, the pressure is on to get it perfect and we rehearse for many, many hours.

The programme always starts with 'Once in Royal David's City' and ends with 'Hark the Herald Angels'. I absolutely love it; all those old favourite carols are so good to sing, and the atmosphere when the whole thing comes together is extraordinary. Various members of the university read the lessons, and there's a full congregation in the chapel for both the filmed and the live broadcasts, so it's a lot of fun.

Inevitably, in the last few rehearsals before filming, tempers get frayed. A couple of days ago Stephen Cleobury, the Director of Music, was particularly annoyed with us because half the choir didn't seem to know what they were doing (though they did). He tore a strip off us and it wasn't fun, but I could sort of understand it – I'd probably have got in a strop if I were in his position. Patch did a good job, during the breaks, of reminding the men to keep up their concentration levels. I think we were all nervous before the actual filming. It's just so important that nothing goes wrong, and in situations like that I'm always worried I'll cough and ruin it. But it's also very exciting to be part of something that's such a national treasure and a part of Christmas for an awful lot of people.

In the end all the strops and nerves and rehearsals paid off and the filming went without a hitch. The only blunder for me was the fact that (due to nerves) I hadn't eaten since the previous evening, so it was lucky that Mum and Dad were in the congregation – afterwards they took me and Patch out for supper.

Now that I've got a bit more time on my hands I'm trying to catch up with work, and talking to Lils quite a lot now. I still really like her, but the fact we are talking so much seems to be getting on her nerves – we broke up because the long distances couldn't work, but now we're making it work, because we're in touch all the time. She does have a point I suppose.

A couple of days ago she wrote an email expanding on some of the things that irritate her about me. Nothing in it really surprised me . . .

She said: 'You are so used to getting your own way that you tell me what to do all the time, like telling me what to wear and not wear. Which is a bit much, especially if we're not even going out. Then, the "I love you but I can still see other people on the side" attitude really annoys me. And you can be so rude sometimes – I know it's all meant to be a joke but then you go too far. And then you get offended when I am even the slightest bit rude or sarcastic back. Finally, you admire Patch so much – he can do no wrong and whatever he says goes. Patch doesn't like my leopard-print coat, so neither do you – and that can be very, very irritating.'

Well, I have to take issue with some of that! For a start, it was me who didn't like the coat, and Patch just happened to agree. And I don't think I'm that rude. But OK, she does have some fair points. I know I am used to getting my own way, though I like to think it's because I'm persuasive rather than spoiled.

I have in fact asked myself if I'm spoiled and I've tried to be honest. I do get a lot of attention, and have a lot of things done for me, because of my illness. And I suppose that's got me used to getting my own way. But, on the other hand, I've never been mollycoddled. My parents always encouraged me to do as much as I possibly could for myself; they didn't wrap me in cotton wool or fuss over me. And that's made me very independent in many ways. So I hope I'm not spoiled, but I'm certainly bearing Lils's comments in mind.

I don't mind Lils being truthful. And she does say that she forgives me for my faults because I'm very romantic. I think I even promised to write a song for her! Meanwhile she bought me an absolutely enormous beanbag. It arrived in the plodge (porter's lodge), where it took up a ridiculous amount of their space and annoyed them all considerably. I couldn't carry it by myself so it had to stay there until I could find help. I got Patch, but he couldn't manage it by himself either. In the end, Patch and a friend of his rolled it back to my room.

When I eventually got the packaging off, I could see it really was an awesome beanbag. Black – and so big that I can lie on it fully stretched out. It takes up half the floor space in my living room. I'll definitely miss it when I'm not in Cambridge.

Mum came up to sort out my stuff for the tour. One of the matrons at King's prep school will be coming along on the trip and will give me a hand, so she came over to go through everything with Mum. She'll make sure I take all my tablets and make up the shakes for me three times a day to keep my calorie intake up. I don't take my night feed along – it's too complicated to set up in a different hotel each night.

After Mum left, I felt I had perhaps been a bit short with her again. She's so used to organising it all for me, but I really wanted to do the packing myself this time. When Mum is packing it reminds me of being back in prep school – but I know that's no excuse for snapping at her and I felt a bit bad after she left. Promised myself I'd call her before we set off.

I love travelling, even though it gets tiring. I did a couple of tours with the choir at Eton – to the USA in 2004 and Australia and New Zealand in 2005 – and before that I toured with King's in Greece, France, Belgium, Holland and Germany.

We flew from Stansted again and had a twenty-kilo baggage allowance per person, which in my case had to include medicines, shakes, nebulisers, two oxygen cylinders, and the size-one cricket bat which I take with me everywhere I go. In addition, each of us older choristers had to take the music for one of the little ones. And I had to fit in clothes too. On tour we wear a dinner jacket or college gown for concerts. I managed to cram it all in eventually, but goodness knows how.

I loved being in Rome. I didn't see Lils because she was already back in England for the holidays, but Patch and I were able to meet up with Miranda, who came over from Paris to see us. We all went for lunch and I had one of the best pizzas I've ever had, followed by superb Italian ice-cream.

In the hotel Patch and I shared a room, which was quite tough on him, because he was trying to study. It wasn't all one-way, though. He had clearly forgotten to pack any socks and kept slyly taking mine. By the time we got back from the tour I had none left!

The good thing about this hotel was that it had a nice wide corridor, perfect for a bit of after-dinner corridor cricket – which is how most of us spend down-time after all the flying and singing. We were very wary of annoying other guests, or breaking windows, apart from one guy (not mentioning any names, Kanag) who clearly had no worries about the windows at all; he hit the ball so hard (and erratically) it went all over the place, bouncing off the walls.

After Rome we headed for Eindhoven in Holland. On this flight the baggage allowance was fifteen kilos, and meanwhile I had somehow gained extra baggage, so my stuff now weighed twenty-five. (Shouldn't have brought that cricket bat.) So Patch and I had to completely re-organise our bags and do a lot of shuffling of my stuff (in addition to the stolen socks) over to his.

After Eindhoven it was on to Amsterdam and our final concert, in front of a very appreciative audience at the stunning Concertgebouw, before flying home.

It was an exhilarating experience singing in such a famous venue, and I was sad to leave it. But ultimately I was very tired and happy to be going home . . .

Patch and I headed straight back to Kent from the airport, both of us pretty exhausted. Mum said what she always says: that I was looking thin. I find it very hard not to lose weight on tour. I can't eat just before I sing, and without the night feeds I need a lot of extra calories during the day, so it's hard to keep my weight stable.

It would probably have been a good idea to rest for a few days after the tour. I knew I was very tired – and heading for hospital again if I didn't slow right down. But we got back a week before Christmas, and there was such a lot of good stuff going on. So I decided to keep going and try to make it through Christmas.

Two days after we got back the choir took part in a huge Christmas Concert in the Albert Hall. I had sung there as a chorister and I remember it being so much fun. And it was this time too – we all had a fantastic night, full of carols and fun songs and laughter. Afterwards I went over to Lils to stay the night and it was great to catch up with her.

The next day my brothers and I went carol singing to raise money for CF research. We get a whole lot of friends together and go every year – we've been doing it for the past five years. Lils came along too and we all met at 11 a.m. outside Marks and Spencer in Fenchurch Street. We always start there, and they usually give us a free lunch in the staff canteen, but this year – to the dismay of several of us, who'd been looking forward to the excellent M&S staff food – they gave us sandwiches. Must be the credit crunch . . .

There were about twenty of us, and we put on a good show and sang all the old favourites. Dad came to say 'hi', because it's quite near where he works. Then we went down to the Burlington Arcade, haunt of the seriously rich. Occasionally we spot a celebrity buying extravagant gifts (I got quite excited a few years back when Edwin van der Sar, the Man U goalkeeper, was around), but sadly there weren't many about this year – though we did see Queen's Brian May walking past.

Afterwards Patch and I headed back to Cambridge because we had a choir concert in Birmingham the next day. Then we had a couple of much-needed days off before the final Christmas run. Patch had to work, but most of the rest of us played a bit of cricket and watched some really bad films, like *Home Alone Two*, and *Not Another Teen Movie*. I also nipped out to get presents for the family and managed to wrap the whole thing up in about twenty minutes – which is a record, even for me. We don't do over-the-top presents in our family, and Christmas shopping is never my idea of fun, but I did want to make a bit of an effort. I went to Borders for books and HMV for DVDs and found presents for Mum, Dad, Miranda and Patch. Chris was getting socks (surprise, surprise), and money that I owe him – but I forgot to buy the socks.

I nipped into the sports shop in town and got a good deal on loads of tennis balls too, which should last me a while. I also bought really lightweight bright-yellow plastic cricket stumps. They're brilliant as I can cart them round to play cricket anywhere.

Took everything home, wrapped all the presents, then cooked a lot of sausages, watched more films, and played more cricket. Bliss.

The next day we choral scholars – we're the only students left in Cambridge now – went to join the staff Christmas lunch in College Hall. We had roast turkey with all the trimmings, which was delicious, before rehearsing for the Christmas Eve service. Afterwards I went to Sainsbury's with a few others to get the food for the Christmas Day breakfast. Traditionally, first-year choral scholars have to cook breakfast for all the choral scholars and their families before the Christmas Day service. We're doing it in my flat this year, because the cooker in Market Hostel, where the other first-years live, is broken. We had a budget of £75, and we blew the lot on masses of sausages, bacon, eggs, bread, beans, tea, coffee and some vegetarian stuff, all of which we carted back to my flat. Lucky, I have *two* fridges – for all my shakes.

In the evening all the choral scholars and the Dean

and Chaplain went to the Chophouse for a meal. You'd have thought no one would have been hungry, after the enormous lunch, but we managed to put away a very substantial dinner too. When we came back some of us played even more cricket well into the night, which was bloody cold, but great fun. You'd think by now some of us should have improved, but no, Kanag is still very uncoordinated.

The next day – Christmas Eve – the men of the choir sang a short fifteen-minute service in the morning for Radio 4 LW, before having a final hour-length practice for the big radio service in the afternoon. This is the second 'Carols from Kings', the service that goes out live on Radio 4/the BBC World Service to 145 million people around the world, and then at 3 p.m. on Christmas Day on BBC Radio 3. That's quite an awesome thought and I think we were all nervous as we didn't want to muck it up. I worked hard on clearing my lungs and warming up my voice beforehand, and by the time of the service I was ready to give it my best shot.

The thing is that people queue for a couple of days just to get into the Christmas Eve service at King's. By the night before there were loads of people queuing outside the porter's lodge and in the morning they let them in to queue in the courtyard. As usual, the choral scholars rustle up a few light-hearted Christmas numbers like 'Rudolf the Red-nosed Reindeer', 'Jingle Bells', 'White Christmas' and so on, which we sang to all the different parts of the queue at lunch to keep them entertained.

The sense of anticipation was enormous, in the congregation and among all of us in the choir. There's something about Christmas that makes everything more mysterious, and this service is, for a lot of people, the essence of Christmas, because it combines the story of Jesus with some very beautiful and uplifting music.

In the end all the rehearsing paid off, and it went without a hitch. I think we all felt pleased, and relieved that it was in the bag.

Mum and Chris came up for it but sadly afterwards they left to go home because they had volunteered to prepare Christmas lunch for the rest of us – that's dedication.

In the evening Dad arrived with Grandpa and Miranda, who came over on Eurostar. It was really wonderful to see her. Grandpa – Dad's father – is still going strong at eighty-two. My grandmother died last year, so he's on his own now, but he's still very active and is a member of the Hampshire Cricket Club. He's a bit deaf, which is a shame because he loves music.

All the choral scholars and staff and relatives had drinks in College Hall, then we watched the TV recording of 'Carols from King's' that we made a couple of weeks ago. And after that we had a dinner of roast partridge. This was immense, as I had never tried it before, but it was delicious – as was the rest of the meal. Even though we were all absolutely stuffed, after dinner we played games involving wrestling, tennis balls and dustbins before Dad, Grandpa and Miranda went off to stay in college guest rooms.

On Christmas Day I got up very early and made breakfast for twenty-five people, with the five other first-years. I was in my usual 'early morning daze', but the guests arrived at 8.30 so the pressure was on and I made sure I was ready. We didn't have enough rings on the hob to do everything at once, so we had to feed people in relays. The place was packed; there were people everywhere. And, of course, the smoke alarm went off – twice – and the porters had to come over quite regularly to make sure everything was running smoothly. But I didn't feel too bad about it – apparently when the third-years did the breakfast two years ago they set off the smoke alarm three times.

We had a conveyor belt of the six of us passing out plates of food, but we had to rush, because we had rehearsal at 9.15 for the service at 11. People didn't get a lot of choice about what they ate. It was too hard trying to take orders, so we just bunged some of everything on each plate and somehow managed to get the lot fed, and the plates shoved in the sink, before rushing over to the chapel to sling on our cassocks and line up looking vaguely angelic.

Dad, Miranda and Grandpa came to the service, which is one of my favourites because there's no TV or recording, so less pressure and we can just enjoy it. Afterwards we all drove home to find Mum cooking a late lunch with Chris, Granny and two of our uncles. There were ten of us around the table and it was a bit of a crush, but we had a massive and brilliant lunch. I really do savour Christmas lunch – and it's lucky I do because I've managed to eat several of them this year.

We did a bit of present-swapping next. Everyone seemed to like what I'd got for them. Last year I bought everyone 10p books from a charity shop and I'm quite put out that they still haven't read them! Patch got a book about *Test Match Special* on BBC4 and Chris got *How to Make Loads of Money in the City*. I thought I got the perfect books. They gave me a golf club – a 3 wood, which I've actually put to good use down on various tees around Kent.

This year Chris didn't get me a present, even though he got everyone else one. My siblings and I are a bit inconsistent with our presents, but even so I was shocked. His excuse was that it was hard to find a present for me. That's feeble – he could have got socks. But then I remembered that I hadn't got him a present either! I had meant to buy him socks and had forgotten. I in fact got a lot of socks from my parents, and Patch got me purple and white King's College socks, while Miranda got me a woolly hat.

A Boy Called Alex was shown again on Christmas afternoon. I was really surprised; I know it got a good audience when it was first shown, but I would never have expected them to repeat it at such a peak viewing time. Then again, it was up against *Doctor Who* ... I felt quite touched it was on, but I didn't actually want to watch it, because it's quite embarrassing watching myself and I've seen it several times before. But Mum and Granny got the deciding vote regardless of me and my brothers' protests. I myself fell asleep after five minutes ...

Actually, I slept for a lot of the next couple of days. Great as all the Christmas concerts and services were, they left me feeling pretty wiped out. I was very chuffed that I'd made it to every single event, but by Boxing Day all I wanted to do was sleep, eat, watch TV and sleep some more.

By the day after Boxing Day my chest was beginning to feel very heavy. It had been going that way for a few days, but as is my way (apparently), I pushed myself to keep going, and then it caught up with me. Mum and Dad suggested it would be a good idea to go into hospital but I didn't agree. However, the next day I made a personal decision to go in as the timing felt good, because it was the holidays. I hoped I could have a couple of weeks of treatment and get back for the start of next term.

The Brompton said they didn't have a spare bed for a couple of days, so I rested at home, and went in on the 29th to be met by the usual battery of tests. My lung function was down to 29 per cent again, so I was back on the intravenous antibiotics and spent the next few days feeling very groggy.

Lils came in and it was really good to see her because we haven't caught up since the carol singing. She invited me to her house for dinner on New Year's Eve and the doctors said I could go, as long as I was back within a couple of hours. Not exactly a typical New Year's Eve for someone my age, but it was lovely of Lils and her mum to ask me. When I arrived we had a really nice dinner with her brother and friends Gigi and Anna before I had to go back to the hospital early – which was annoying, but it was nice to get out.

I got back to the hospital by 10 p.m. and called a few friends, and the hospital staff did their best to make it festive for all of us. But parties in hospital are never going to be *quite* the same as parties out of hospital, and I was the youngest one in the adult unit by quite a bit, so couldn't help wishing that I was somewhere with just a bit more buzz to it. At midnight itself I counted down with the nurses who were on duty before heading off to watch highlights of the Boxing Day test between Australia and South Africa.

January 2009

My life owes a lot to music

The beginning of a new year and the biggest thing ahead of me is the *Matthew Passion* concert. It's only three months away, which suddenly feels alarmingly close, so I decided to use my time in hospital to really get to grips with the score.

I've listened to it many times now, so my next step is to work through the written score, getting to know it and making decisions about how I want each section to sound. I've been given a huge conductors' score by my parents, about two foot square and 300 pages long, with the entire score in incredible detail. It's immensely complex – not just because of the length, but because of the scale. Both the choir and the orchestra have to be split into two separate halves for the performance. It's more dramatically intense than the *Magnificat*, but also more reflective. I've also got a book on conducting that Ralph gave me, written by the renowned conductor Sir Adrian Boult. It's very precise, right down to the timings of the tea breaks!

I've been singing every part to myself as I go through it. I can't conduct it properly if I don't know all the parts. And I'm enjoying myself; the more I get to know it, the more I understand its depths and layers and brilliance.

I'm thinking about how to organise the rehearsals. I'll only have five days of rehearsals – Ralph has arranged to have them in Westminster School, where there will be space because the kids will have gone home for the Easter holidays. So I've got to make the most of every minute and try to ensure there aren't too many of the musicians sitting around for too long.

The news on the fund-raising side is really good. There's a way to go, but money is steadily coming in from supporters who want to see the concert happen, and the tickets are selling fast. The most expensive tickets are £150, for people who want to give an extra donation. It's a lot to ask, but a fair number of them have sold.

I'm aware that there's a lot of expectation riding on me, and I want to deliver. This is my chance to show a wider audience that I can do it, musically. I want to prove myself, and I don't want any concessions. I'd be very upset if anyone imagined I'd been given this chance just because I have a disease, and that I wasn't really up to it. I'm pretty sure I'm good enough to do it on musical merit, and I know Ralph believes I am, or he wouldn't be putting in so much effort. He wouldn't want me to be seen as a performing monkey, any more than I would – we'd both be horrified if people thought, 'Oh, look at him, isn't he good? He's so young and, boo hoo, he's ill.' I never feel 'look at me' when I'm in front of an audience. What I feel is 'listen to the music', and that's what I'm working towards – I want the audience to be totally absorbed by the music.

Nevertheless, I'm very aware that some parts of the *Matthew Passion* will be harder to hold together than others. The most difficult chorus of all is a glorious one at the end of the first half, 'O Mankind Bewail Your Destiny'. It's one of Bach's most uplifting passages, extraordinary and intricate, and it needs every performer to really be on their mettle and listen to one another and follow the conductor closely, because the timing is vital. I know it's going to be a bit of a pain to keep together, so that everyone comes in on time.

Bach's music, for me, is the kind that convinces you there is something greater than yourself. It's certainly beyond words – my words, anyway. I know how deeply it makes me feel, but all I can say to someone about it is 'listen'. To me, music is the most powerful utterance that mankind has discovered. It can't be explained, it simply is, and I am grateful for it every day of my life.

While I've been immersing myself in the masterpiece, the time in hospital has passed and I'm finally getting better. I've had to break off from the *Matthew*

Passion, though, to look at some of next term's assign-ments, which came through on email. These days there's no escaping tutors. We're doing pre-fifteenth-century sacred music next term which I'm not too excited about. I suppose it all goes back to being a chorister and being indoctrinated by older boys into hating 'chod' – a term used to describe a lot of pre-seventeenth-century music.

A week after I went into hospital it was Mum's birthday. It was a Tuesday and she was teaching, so I didn't see her until the next day. She was due to come in at 10 a.m., so I nipped out and got a bus up the road to where there's an M&S and bought her some flowers. I got back just after she arrived, to find her looking for me. She said, 'Oh Alexander, you really shouldn't have gone out', but she was very pleased with the flowers. I know I *still* don't do enough for her, but I try!

Chris and Dad have been in to see me lots, and so has Lils, though she's about to go back to Rome. I'm going to miss her; it's been really good having her around. We still spend most of our time swap-ping insults. Even when I'm lying on my hospital bed, we are merciless with one another.

By the time I'd been in hospital for ten days I was feeling desperate to get back to Cambridge. Term was due to start a couple of days later and I just wanted to get there and get on with some work and catch up with friends. Hospital is no substitute for real life. So

I was really happy when the doctor arrived and said that as I had made a big improvement – my lung function was back up to 40 per cent – I could leave the next day and finish the course of antibiotics back at college.

Mum promised to come and get me as early as possible and I spent the evening banging a tennis ball against the wall in my room, venting my frustration at having to wait.

I really did feel sorry for Mum the following day. She got up at 4.30 a.m. to get to the Brompton by 7, and when she finally arrived there was no space – disabled or otherwise – so she drove round and round looking for one, and the parking attendant just kept telling her to keep trying. She was so stressed that she burst into tears – and it takes a lot to make Mum do that. Finally she got one, and then, after all that, we had to wait until 2 p.m. for the doctors to let me go.

After that we crawled up the motorway with the surrounding landscape cloaked in a spectacular hoar frost. After we got back to King's, Mum stayed on to help me unpack, got some supplies for me from Sainsbury, and cooked me dinner of lamb chops and roast potatoes with a very nice Yorkshire pud. I don't know how she made it, but it was delicious. She left at about 8 p.m. for the drive home. A really long day for her, and I was pretty worried about how tired she would be the following one.

Then, on my first day back, I hit problems. First of all my scooter stopped working. And then I couldn't get the antibiotics into my portacath – normally I just stick the syringe into the line attached to the porta-cath, but that day something went wrong; it hurt a fair bit and the drugs just wouldn't go in. I realised the line was somehow blocked. I tried to flush the line, to clear it, but it didn't work, so I rang Mum, who said to ring Vicky, who said to ring Papworth. After a minor communication crisis, I eventually got through to the consultant, who told me to come straight in. The porters got me a taxi and Patch came with me to the porter's lodge. I wouldn't let him come with me to hospital, though; he's got lots to do and, contrary to his concerns, I knew I'd be fine on my own.

In hospital they were great. Took out the line, cleared it and put it back, and I was back in college in about three hours.

The next day was Sunday, so my parents came up to visit and Dad fixed the scooter – it was just a loose wire which must have got knocked when the battery was changed.

After that, I got back into a normal routine. Back to choir duties a couple of days after term started, and back to the library, as I had loads of essays to catch up on. Mum helped by arriving with a new microwave and some ready meals. Good move, as it'll be a lot easier for me to just heat up a meal, and it should give the porters and the fire brigade a break too. The thing is, Mum also asked me if I was OK with the microwave being my birthday present (er, I don't think you're going to get away with that one, Mum . . .).

In the meantime Ralph got in touch to say the *Matthew Passion* team has raised £19,000 of the £25,000 they need, and that tickets are still selling really well. Everyone believes we'll make it, and I'm so grateful for all the hard work that's gone into it.

In the next few weeks I'm hoping to go and see one or two well-known conductors to get insight into the work from those who know it inside out. In the end, I'll be eternally grateful for all the advice and ideas I get.

The 30th of January was my nineteenth birthday. Nineteenth birthdays are usually non-events compared to 18ths and 21sts, but I did value this birthday, because it was the first one in a while that I wasn't in hospital for!

The senior scholars in the choir, including Patch, were doing a concert in Peterborough, so I went out for a curry with some of the other choral scholars and then had a few people back to my rooms for a 'wine and cricket' party (it'll catch on, trust me) afterwards. And I actually got some great presents! Lizzy, a first-year friend of mine – and one of Coll Reg's most dedicated followers – gave me some socks. The nice thing was that she'd drawn the first two bars of the *Matthew Passion* on the pink ones and the first two bars of 'Wintereisse', my favourite Schubert song-cycle, on the blue ones. Clever. And another friend gave me an old-fashioned bike horn for my scooter. Can't wait to annoy every tutor in earshot by squeezing it as I break every porter-imposed speed limit through college. Patch came by after the Peterborough gig and joined us for a bit. In the end we all stayed up much too late, and once they'd gone I realised the living room was a complete tip. I was too knackered to tidy it, though, and instead slumped on the bed after having one of the most enjoyable birthdays for ages.

On the following Sunday my parents arrived with a second-hand table and bench for my living room, which was brilliant as I really needed a table. At the moment everything gets dumped on the floor. Goodness knows how they got it in the car, though. They took me out for a steak at lunchtime and in the afternoon it started snowing. By evening it was quite deep and the whole of the back lawn at King's was white. A few hours after evensong most of the college came on to the lawn for a massive snowball fight. Snow is a rare treat; I can only remember it once or twice during my childhood when it was this heavy, so I wasn't going to pass up the chance now.

February 2009

We all get inspiration

It was arranged that I should meet the renowned Russian pianist and conductor Vladimir Ashkenazy, so at the beginning of this month I caught the train from Cambridge and we met over a drink, in a London hotel. He is someone I admire enormously. I have quite a few of his recordings; he is extraordinary, and to watch him is to see a master at work.

He is now over seventy and he has been on the world stage for more than fifty years. Starting off as a pianist, he showed extraordinary talent as a child and went on to win many international piano competitions. Later on he branched out into conducting, and since then he has worked with orchestras around the world, including seven years as conductor of the Royal Philharmonic Orchestra. Today he is chief conductor of the Sydney Symphony, as well as being conductor laureate of several orchestras, including the Philharmonia, which is based in London.

A year ago I met Nigel Black, who is the principal

horn of the Philharmonia. He was incredibly nice and took a lot of interest in me, and he was one of the people who arranged a concert at St James's Palace in aid of CF, at which both Ashkenazy and I were due to play. The concert was to have been this month, and I was very excited – and nervous – about the performance as well as the idea of meeting Vladimir Ashkenazy himself. But then the concert had to be cancelled because the funding couldn't be raised because of the economic climate. Credit crunch again . . .

I was very disappointed and thought my chance to meet Ashkenazy had gone – until I received another call from Nigel Black, who said that Ashkenazy was coming to London anyway, as he had a concert with the Philharmonia the day after our concert was to have been held. Nigel told me then that Ashkenazy had invited me to go and meet him for a drink.

We can't usually miss evensong for anything other than illness, without official permission. So I had to ask Stephen Cleobury, the Director of Music, if I could go. He insisted I go to the afternoon practice, but said I could go after that, and miss the actual service. So after practice I got the train down to London and went along to the Berkeley Hotel in Knightsbridge, where we were due to meet at 7 p.m.

I got there twenty minutes early, at 6.40, because I wanted to make a fairly good impression. It was a very grand hotel and when I walked in it was full of smartly dressed couples waiting to go in for dinner. I spotted Nigel and Ashkenazy talking over to one side, but they didn't see me, so I turned round and went out again because I was so nervous. Good start. I paced up and down outside for a bit, thinking about what I wanted to say, and then went back in.

I was still feeling extremely nervous, but needn't have worried as Ashkenazy put me at ease straight-away, telling me how pleased he was that I was able to come, and how much he had heard about me. He had just finished a long rehearsal and I could see he was tired, but we chatted for an hour and he asked about my music and what I want to do. There was no piano in the hotel so I couldn't play for him (which might have been just as well), but he was very encour-aging and that meant a lot to me.

He told me of his constant desire to practise the piano – not just his current repertoire, but also tech-nical exercises like scales, which is something I should definitely aim to do more of.

He had lots of funny anecdotes, and he talked about the possibility of us finally doing the concert together later in the year. As we parted, we all agreed to do our best to work together to make this happen, which will be fantastic if it comes off.

When I got back to Cambridge, Patch wanted to know all about it. I also phoned Lils and chatted for a bit. We always end up talking for far too long. Even when I don't want to talk to her, I want to talk to her. Make any sense? Nope, thought not.

A week or so after meeting Ashkenazy, I was back at Papworth for a meeting I'd much rather not have had. It was MOT time again and the results were a tad annoying. The consultant did say I'd done better than expected since my last stint in hospital in October, so that was encouraging. But my lung function is slightly down and I've lost a fair bit of weight. My Body Mass Index was 17.4 last time; now it's 17.0. Basically it needs to be up to 20. Hopefully then Mum won't say I look as if a puff of wind will knock me down. I know I'm stronger than everyone thinks, but don't think anybody believes me!

Actually I have been a bit slack sometimes regarding my night feeds, and the consultant was quite firm in telling me I can't afford to miss any. I know he's right, because I can't actually eat any more than I already do. I *try* to eat more, but I feel full very quickly, and once you feel full it's hard to make yourself eat more. And anyway, sometimes I'm just too tired to eat.

The doctor said my lungs are in a pretty poor shape – it's becoming standard hearing that now. He asked me if I'd like to see the CT scan they did last autumn. I declined the offer – I know my lungs aren't good; I don't need to see it in detail.

He was fairly blunt and said, 'You're worse than you think you are.' With respect to him, I don't agree.

I know what's going on in my own body better than anyone, regardless of all the figures doctors put in front of me. He said he thought I might need some extra antibiotics soon, but agreed with my plan to wait and see how I get on.

Prompted by my ever-cautious mum, I asked him if he thought I'd be able to go on the eight-day choir tour to Singapore in July. He said that I needed to get better first, and that if the trip were tomorrow, he'd be extremely worried about letting me go.

After our meeting with him, we saw the dietician. She wants me to take 'booster shots' of a very high-calorie drink called 'Calogen'. They put 125 calories into a 30 ml drink, and I would need at least three a day to make a difference. I asked if I could wait until the summer to start them, and she said, 'There's no point doing this when you're dead.' Hmmm ... I think she's saying she wants me to take them now, so fine, I will.

They also offered me a new nebuliser treatment. I'm actually happy with the one I have, but they think the new one might give me more help with shifting the mucus in my lungs. Again I asked if I could start this one in the summer, and they reluctantly agreed, but suggested it would be better to try it now.

My problem is that I don't like change when it comes to my health – I'd rather stick with the treatments I'm used to. I think I've got a bit of a block about new treatments, and always have to be talked into trying them. I guess it's the same thing as taking my tablets. When you prefer to ignore your illness, focusing on the treatments is hard.

Anyway, the upshot (for the doctors anyway) was that I will take the booster shots, make sure I have my night feed, and go back for another check-up in a month. I'm basically pretty pleased because I escaped being admitted. I desperately want to get through to the end of term, and the *Matthew Passion* concert, before I go into hospital again.

Things are hotting up quite a bit for the 'MattPash' (now my nickname for the work). I've been asked to appear on BBC *Breakfast Time* and to give several newspaper interviews in the build-up to the concert. There's quite a bit of interest, which is good, though it also ups the pressure. I've already done a piece for the *Daily Mail*'s *Weekend* magazine which appeared a few weeks ago, and next up it's the *Independent* and *The Sunday Times*.

March 2009

A month of Passion

Another very special meeting became a reality this month when I met Sir David Willcocks. A distinguished conductor, organist and Director of the King's College Choir from 1957 to 1974, he will be ninety this year, but he's still in good health. He has remained in Cambridge, and lives very near my old school. Ralph knows David, so kindly arranged the meeting.

Sir David has what I would call presence, and when he speaks, you find yourself listening to every word. I can certainly see how he had full command of a choir and orchestra.

Sir David has conducted the *Matthew Passion* many times, so I was hoping to pick up some tips from him, and it was in fact a very interesting meeting. He had lots of stories about his experiences conducting the MattPash, and also gave me some very useful advice. He was keen that I made sure the soloists are not too overworked and talked about how much planning is involved in rehearsing. He also showed me a sample rehearsal schedule which he uses, and that was really helpful. I can see that you've got to manage it so that everyone has enough rehearsal time, and enough breaks, but not *so* much time that they're just sitting around. It's a question of careful planning and quite a bit of juggling.

I had two hours with him in the end, and he talked quite a bit about his life, which was fascinating. At the end of our time together he wished me luck and said he'd be at the concert, which was incredibly supportive of him – though just a touch daunting for me!

I seem to be sleeping, eating and breathing the MattPash at the moment. And, as luck would have it, a performance was put on in the Trinity College chapel by Clare College, just days after my meeting with Sir David. The tickets were on sale at the Corn Exchange, but unfortunately by the time I got there they were all sold – except the £5 standing ones. My chest wasn't feeling too good by now – in fact, I had to take a fistful of paper towels along because I was coughing so much. I knew I couldn't stand for the whole three hours, so when I got there I said I was a bit deaf and asked whether I could sit on the steps leading up to the Provost's chair. A girl sitting in the chorus suddenly piped up, 'Why don't you sit in the Provost's chair until he comes?' So I did – but then the Provost arrived and he didn't look too pleased.

Luckily I did manage to find a seat. I had considered bringing my score along and writing notes on it during the performance, but I'd have felt like a bit of a gimp doing that, so I didn't take it in the end, and scribbled notes on my programme. And, in any case, I felt pretty unwell during the first part of the performance, so I just shut my eyes and listened. I woke up a bit in the second part and paid more attention.

Overall I thought it was a good performance, but there were some things I intend to do very differently. These are mainly to do with the tempos, but some are issues of stage management – that is, where everybody is playing/singing.

The following day I had a call from Ralph to say that the MattPash concert is now sold out. Not only that, but enough money had been raised to pay for the performance and give a substantial donation to CF research. That was great news, and it really lifted my spirits. I had been feeling a bit annoyed, because despite my best efforts I knew my health wasn't brilliant at that point, but knowing that everything was in place felt encouraging. So many people had put in effort to make it happen; I wasn't going to let them down.

Lils flew over for the weekend just after I got this news, and that cheered me up too. She was her usual chatty self, but I was actually quite annoyed with her on the Friday night because she was meant to come and hear me in evensong. *Somehow* she managed to miss her train up from London. But I eventually forgave her and we went to the curry house with Robbie and his girlfriend Gabby, and Dave and Kanag. After that we went to Chet – the Chetwin Society meeting – which is the fortnightly meeting of the choral scholars. Lils enjoyed it, although she said that essentially it was a glorified lads' piss up – the only difference being that it's been going for many years and is all conducted in a reasonably formal tone. I can't argue with her on that one.

On Saturday I had to rehearse for a concert with the choir, so Lils went for a walk and did some shopping. When I got back she told me she'd then tried – and failed – to tidy my room, which, I have to agree, is a real tip.

That evening she came to the concert, which was a magnificent celebration of Mendelssohn as 2009 was the 200th anniversary of his birth, and afterwards we had dinner with a couple of our friends. It was a really good evening (Lils did complain I wasn't eating enough), but that night I felt really ill and barely slept for coughing – so neither of us got much sleep. The next morning Lils didn't want to leave me in what was clearly not good shape, and ended up missing her train. Dedication. She then changed her flight to Monday and we went for lunch in the town. After an hour of nagging that I still wasn't eating enough, we sat by the river eating some homemade fudge until she got a taxi to the station. Lils eventually got back to London in the evening, then caught her flight to Rome the next morning. I, meanwhile, had crashed out on my bed, feeling completely exhausted.

On the Monday morning Mum arrived to take me to Papworth. I had called her because we both knew I needed some intravenous antibiotics. I hoped that the doctors might let me stay in my flat and take the antibiotics there. I really, really didn't want to be admitted to hospital, but when I got there they insisted that I stay. Ultimately, there wasn't a lot I could do. I knew I wasn't in great shape, and with the MattPash now less than three weeks away, I absolutely had to get a bit better.

I spent a week in Papworth, which was just about alright, although I'd rather have been in the Brompton. I had far fewer visitors at Papworth – only my mum in fact – but it was good to have a rest and, while the antibiotics pumped round my system, I listened to the MattPash again and finalised my ideas for the concert.

Nevertheless I was still bloody annoyed. There I was stuck in hospital and the rest of the choral scholars were setting off on a south of England tour that I really wanted to go on. At the very least I had planned to make at least part of the tour, before heading back for the MattPash rehearsals. I still hoped I might make one or two of the concerts if I could get out of hospital in time, but in the end, even though they let me go back to my flat after a week, they refused to let me join the tour.

It was *so* frustrating. I felt I wasn't as bad as they thought I was, and did my utmost to persuade the doctors to let me go. I was certain that if they re-tested me, the results would be better than they expected. But the doctors were adamant, and ulti-mately I reluctantly accepted the verdict.

It was really quiet back at my flat in King's, as there was hardly anyone around. I caught up on a bit of work – and tried not to think about the fact that if I hadn't got ill, I would now be on tour with the others.

But I also knew my voice wasn't up to singing, and I wouldn't have wanted to let the choir down – or Patch – by giving a sub-standard performance.

As it was, I went down to Dorset to see one of the concerts, and meet with another famous conductor, Sir John Elliot Gardiner. He has been conducting since he was fifteen; he was a student at King's and, while he was there, founded the Monteverdi choir. Later on came two orchestras – the English Baroque Soloists and the Orchestre Révolutionnaire et Romantique. After conducting orchestras and choirs all over the world, I knew he'd have some interesting things to say about the MattPash.

On the day I was meeting him I had got up really, really early and caught the train from

Cambridge down to Gillingham in Dorset, and I was so pleased that Sir John talked to me – at length – about different aspects of performing the *Matthew Passion*. The main element we discussed was the layout of the performers on the stage, a part I admittedly hadn't put too much thought into. He also lent me a new book about every aspect of both the *St Matthew* and *St John Passions*, which would turn out to be really interesting reading for the train journey back.

After lunch with Sir John, I caught the train to Beaulieu where seven of Coll Reg were singing in a concert. After catching up with Patch, and watching the concert in the beautiful thirteenth-century abbey, I got the train back to London far too late. But somewhere along the line (no pun intended) – I think it was Andover – I had a really silly accident. There was a tannoy announcement that the train was being divided, and if you wanted to go to London you had to be in the front half. I was in the back, so I realised I needed to get off and run up the platform to the front in order to be on the right bit of the train. Running in the dark, laden down by a ridiculously heavy bag, somehow or other I tripped and fell, gashing my leg quite badly. Thankfully, I still made it on to the train, but when I got to London I found I had missed my connection to Cambridge – which was in fact the last train that night.

I knew my brother Chris would give me a bed for

the night, but as it happened I was quite lucky to find him at all, because he'd been away for a few days. As luck would have it (for me at least), we both ended up at his front door at exactly the same time – 12.30 a.m. Had it been a day earlier, I'm not sure what I would have done as I didn't really have a plan B. The prospect of sleeping on the pavement wasn't entirely appealing.

After catching up with Chris, I travelled back to Cambridge the next day, decidedly shattered, and very much in need of a couple of days' rest while I completed my antibiotics. And a couple of days *were* all I had – because the MattPash rehearsals were due to begin later that week.

April 2009

A night to remember

Rehearsals for the MattPash began on Wednesday, 1 April, in Westminster School. Mum drove me from Cambridge down to London the night before, where I was going to stay with Lils's family, who had generously offered to put me up all week. That made life a lot easier, and it was great to see Lils, who was back from Rome for Easter.

I arrived on the first morning of rehearsals feeling a little nervous because I knew how critical that first day would be. For the first three days it was only the choir rehearsing, before the orchestra and soloists came together with the choir for the last two days. I knew it was important that I pitch things right, as I was working alongside people I hadn't worked with before. I wanted to make sure that they had confidence in me musically, and that they could trust my stewardship.

Of course, my job was made easier by the fact that all the musicians were professional and highly committed. They listened attentively, followed, interpreted, and were in all senses a joy to work with. Ralph was an able assistant conductor, always there to take over if I needed him, but I'm relieved to say I never did. He sat at the back and talked to me in the breaks, and I asked him how he felt it was going. He was always encouraging and supportive, telling me that I was doing just fine, so that, along with the great response from the singers, really calmed my nerves.

We were singing the MattPash in its original German, but unfortunately my German pronunciation isn't that great. Mercifully, there was a girl in the Rodolfus Choir who could speak German fluently, and she was brilliant in helping us to perfect our vowels and consonants.

In terms of tempi, I played around with speeds in the first few rehearsals, but at the third one I set the speeds I wanted right from the start, so that everyone would be in no doubt. When conducting, for me less is more, and grand gestures aren't any more effective than subtle, economical ones. I've always given smaller gestures, but I also try to keep my meaning very clear.

It was pretty tiring work, but at the same time incredibly enjoyable, and by the end of the first day I felt we had all made a good start. And for the next four days it was just a question of keeping up the pace of learning we had achieved during that first day. Rehearsing the luscious chorales and magnificent double choruses proved the most joyful as I directed from the piano – a place where I felt most in control. We rehearsed for several hours each day, so by the time I got back to Lils's house each night I was absolutely shattered. Her mum kindly laid on a nice supper each evening, but I was almost too tired to eat – and during the rehearsals I was so absorbed that thoughts of food didn't even enter my head. Ralph would thrust a Twix in my hand every now and then, but I didn't eat my usual quota. Even so, I was surprised to find that by the time I reached the performance itself I had lost three kilos. Not good.

On the Saturday (which was the only full day of rehearsal with the orchestra) the rehearsal went smoothly, but by the end I was feeling really agitated by my lack of control – or, at least, what I *perceived* to be a lack of control. All the members of the orchestra were really warm and did everything I asked of them, but I just don't think my own concentration was what it could have been.

Then again, the intensity of those rehearsals is hard to describe. For five days I didn't think about anything else at all. I didn't notice the weather, listen to a news bulletin, or think about the clothes I was putting on each day (something that was mercilessly picked upon by a few members of Rods). And although I knew I was tired and my chest was not in a great state, I didn't really think about my health. I knew I would get through it, no matter what, and I put everything I had into bringing all the musicians together in what I hoped would be an emotional performance.

When we finally got to the day of the concert itself, I was reasonably happy with how it had all come together. We had one final rehearsal that morning – it was Sunday, 5 April – and all went well considering the understandable tiredness of everyone involved. But of course with live performance anything can happen, so I was tightly wired.

When I peered out into the hall and saw well over 700 people taking their seats, I felt slightly overwhelmed. But once the musicians had taken their places and I walked out to the podium, I was focused on the music and nothing else.

The first half was going OK, and I felt calm and in control, until the complex chorus just before the end of that half – 'Oh Mankind Bewail Your Destiny'. In rehearsals I had kept every element – strings, wind, continuous and chorus – rigidly in time, but towards the end of this colossal section I was feeling slightly worried that I wasn't really holding everything together. However, it was only momentary, and I knew many people in the audience probably hadn't noticed. But *I* knew, and certainly every other musician would have known, that a mistake had been made.

I was not happy. In fact, I felt damn annoyed and headed back to my dressing room. I was sitting there, trying not to dwell on what had happened, when

Chris walked in. He reassured me that the mistakes were so small that hardly anyone would have noticed, and told me that I now needed to get myself back in a positive frame of mind for the second half of the performance. But for a little while I felt that the whole thing had been spoiled, and I didn't know how I would carry on.

Then Ralph arrived. Seeing how upset I was, he said, 'What would you say to another performer about to go on for a second half after what they'd perceived to be a big mistake? You'd say, "It doesn't matter, look forward, concentrate on the glorious music to come." Well, Alex, that's what you've got to say to yourself now.' He smiled and left me to have a few minutes on my own before I went back on.

As I sat there quietly, I realised that what both Ralph and Chris had said to me had helped. I couldn't afford to get into a state; I needed to look ahead and focus on being calmly in control for the second half. In the end, I managed to get myself together. I went back out, and the second half went well.

At the end of the three-hour performance, the audience rose to their feet and applauded for what I later learned had been five whole minutes. They just didn't seem to want to let us go. It was a damn good feeling.

When I got back to my dressing room I felt sick. I think it was just that I'd put in so much effort to bring it all together and keep myself focused that I hadn't noticed I wasn't well. I found myself retching, and when Mum came in to see me she was really concerned.

I promised her I'd go to hospital the next day, but that night I wanted to celebrate. Mum told me that Sir David Willcocks had been impressed with my conducting – I was delighted by that. I went to thank Ralph and all the musicians; and then Chris, Miranda, Lils and I, along with a few other friends, went out for a pizza and on to the pub. Not sure how I managed it but I did, and despite feeling shattered I was very happy.

I expected that in the morning I would be back in the Brompton, and I was, with all kinds of warnings about low blood sugar and low blood oxygen and poor lung function. I knew I'd probably be there for a few weeks this time, and I was. But at that moment, it didn't matter. Thanks to the many amazing musicians, the evening was a resounding success and certainly one of the highlights of my life so far.

Afterword

by Ralph Allwood

Most musicians come to the *Matthew Passion* quite a bit later on in life, because it's such a big piece. But I knew that Alex was capable of conducting it, and as time is of the essence for him, I felt it was important for him to go ahead.

Alex's story is a vivid and touching one, and there were a great many people who wanted to see the concert realised and who worked hard to make it happen.

Despite the obvious challenges involved, I felt so certain that Alex would rise to meet them that, although I was assistant conductor and would have taken over if Alex had been unable to perform, I hadn't even prepared the score for myself. I knew I wouldn't be needed.

He was clearly musically in charge from the outset, and all the players recognised that and responded. There's a very subtle electricity that connects conductors and performers. The performers decide early on whether they can relate to the conductor, and it was clear that in Alex's case they could.

Alex is a good conductor not because his gestures are particularly elegant – they aren't, but that will improve! He is effective because he knows exactly what he wants others to give the music, and feels it passionately. He can make clear to the performers the basics of his approach to a particular piece of music. This was certainly the case with the *Matthew Passion*.

What sets Alex apart from others is that when he is performing he is able to focus on what lifts him, the music, and is only conscious of the here and now, and not the past or the future. Alex teaches the rest of us how absurd self-pity is. He raises our spirits because his own are almost always so high. And he reminds us that, to quote Anthony Burgess, 'wedged as we are between two eternities of idleness, there is no excuse for being idle now.'